W9-DBT-196

**Edited by
Robert Dunstan**

ABNORMAL LABORATORY RESULTS

MCGRAW-HILL BOOK COMPANY Sydney

New York San Francisco Auckland Bogotá Caracas
Lisbon London Madrid Mexico City Milan Montreal
New Delhi San Juan Singapore Tokyo Toronto

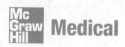

Reprinted 2004

© 2001 Commonwealth Government of Australia: Material published originally in *Abnormal Laboratory Results* in 1987 and in issues of *Australian Prescriber* (since 1989)
© McGraw-Hill Australia Pty Limited: New material
Illustrations and design © 2001 McGraw-Hill Book Company Australia Pty Limited
Additional owners of copyright material are credited in on-page credits.

National Library of Australia Cataloguing-in-Publication data:

Abnormal laboratory results.

ISBN 0 074 70926 7.

1   Diagnosis, Laboratory—Evaluation.
2.   Diagnostic errors.
3.   Clinical chemistry. I. Dunstan, Robert A.

616.0756

Published in Australia by
McGraw-Hill Australia Pty Limited
Level 2, 82 Waterloo Road, North Ryde NSW 2113, Australia
Publishing Manager: Meiling Voon
Production Editor: Megan Lowe
Editor: Joy Window
Interior and Cover Design: Jenny Pace Design
Illustrator: Alan Laver, Shelly Communications
Typeset in Sabon by Jenny Pace Design
Printed on 80gsm woodfree by Pantech, Hong Kong

Foreword

A bewildering array of laboratory tests are available to today's health professionals. There is more to these tests than ticking a box on a request form and looking at the normal range of results. To provide more detail about commonly ordered tests *Australian Prescriber* runs a series called 'Abnormal laboratory results'. Although this may seem an odd topic for a journal mainly concerned with drugs, laboratory tests have an important role in therapeutics.

All the articles from the series were published in a booklet in 1987. This booklet was very popular and although it has long been out of print people still enquire about obtaining a copy. Many more articles have been published in the ensuing years and the millennium seemed an appropriate time to collect them together. This new edition therefore contains all the articles which have been published since the 'Abnormal laboratory results' series began in 1978. The articles have all been updated to include recent advances. In most cases the original authors revised their own papers, although finding these people has involved some detective work.

Compiling all these articles was beyond the resources of *Australian Prescriber*. The Executive Editorial Board is therefore grateful to Dr Robert Dunstan for taking on the responsibility for producing the book and to McGraw-Hill for recognising the need for this publication.

Abnormal Laboratory Results will be of interest to all health professionals and useful background reading for students. It will be complemented by the continued publication of new articles in the *Australian Prescriber* series.

Dr John S. Dowden
Editor, *Australian Prescriber*
Canberra
www.australianprescriber.com

Contents

Preface

Medical laboratory results play a vital role in the diagnosis of disease and the monitoring of treatment. However, pathology testing is becoming increasingly complex and evidence-based medicine is contributing to a rapidly expanding knowledge base. For those in the health care industry, staying abreast of the growth in pathology is becoming increasingly difficult.

In 1987 the journal *Australian Prescriber* published a book titled *Abnormal Laboratory Results*. The book contained 14 articles that had been previously published in the journal in a series of the same name. Since that time *Australian Prescriber* has continued to publish articles in that series and now 37 have been published.

McGraw-Hill approached me in 2000 to edit a second compilation of these articles. I have been able to gather together 31 of the original 37. All of the original authors, with one exception, have been given the opportunity to update their original articles. Where necessary or appropriate this has been done. One of the articles (Chapter 25 'HIV testing in Australia') is such an extensive revision that it should be considered a new article that has not been through the *Australian Prescriber* review process. This book is by no means a comprehensive coverage of laboratory tests and procedures but rather a reflection of the articles covered in *Australian Prescriber*.

Robert A. Dunstan

Contributors

T. I. Robertson MD, FRACP, FRCP   Chapter 1
Former Visiting Physician
Westmead Hospital, Sydney, Australia

C. G. Fraser BSc, PhD, FAACB   Chapter 2
Clinical Leader
Department of Biochemical Medicine
Ninewells Hospital & Medical School, Dundee, Scotland

G. M. Kellerman   Chapter 3
Emeritus Professor of Medical Biochemistry,
University of Newcastle, VMO in Clinical Chemistry
Hunter Area Pathology Service, Newcastle, Australia

T. H. Mathew MBBS, FRACP   Chapter 4
Associate Professor and Director
Renal Unit
The Queen Elizabeth Hospital, Woodville, Australia

G. S. Stokes   Chapter 5
Professor and Head
Hypertension Unit, Cardiology
Royal North Shore Hospital, Sydney, Australia

E. P. MacCarthy   Chapter 5
Head
Hypertension Unit, University of Cincinnati Medical Centre
Cincinnati, Ohio, United States of America

R. G. Larkins Chapter 6
Professor and Dean
Faculty of Medicine, Dentistry and Health Sciences
University of Melbourne, Melbourne, Australia

P. Nestel AO, MD, FRACP, FTSE Chapter 7
Professor
Baker Medical Research Institute and Heart Centre
Alfred Hospital, Melbourne, Australia

A. M. Dart BA, BM, BCh, DPhil, FRCP Chapter 8
Professor
Alfred Hospital and Baker Medical Research Institute
Melbourne, Australia

C. Reid BA, Dip Ed, MSc, DPhil Chapter 8
Alfred Hospital and Baker Medical Research Institute
Melbourne, Australia

G. L. Jennings MBBS, MD, MRCP, FRACP, FRCP Chapter 8
Professor
Alfred Hospital and Baker Medical Research Institute
Melbourne, Australia

R. A. J. Conyers BSc(Hons), MBBS, MAACB, FRCPA, Chapter 8
DPhil
Department of Clinical Biochemistry
The Alfred Hospital, Melbourne, Australia

E. M. Nicholls MBBS, MD, FAFOM Chapter 8
Alfred Hospital and Baker Medical Research Institute
Melbourne, Australia

B. T. Emmerson AO, MD, PhD, FRACP Chapter 9
Emeritus Professor
Department of Medicine, University of Melbourne
Honorary Research Consultant
Princess Alexandra Hospital, Woolloongabba, Australia

L. W. Powell AC, FTSE, MD, PhD, DUniv, FRACP, FRCP   Chapter 10
Professor
Department of Medicine, University of Queensland and
Queensland Institute of Medical Research
Royal Brisbane Hospital, Brisbane, Australia

M. L. Bassett MB, ChB, MD, FRACP   Chapter 10
Associate Professor, Canberra Clinical School,
University of Sydney
Director of Gastroenterology
Canberra Hospital, Canberra, Australia

W. G. E. Cooksley MD, FRACP   Chapter 10
Professor and Director
Clinical Research Centre
Royal Brisbane Hospital Research Foundation,
Brisbane, AUSTRALIA

S. K. Gan MBBS, FRACP   Chapter 11
Clinical Research Fellow
Diabetes and Metabolism Research Program
Garvan Institute of Medical Research
St Vincent's Hospital, Sydney, Australia

D. J. Chisholm AO, MBBS, FRACP   Chapter 11
Professor and Head
Diabetes and Metabolism Research Program
Garvan Institute of Medical Research
St Vincent's Hospital, Sydney, Australia

G. Jones MBBS, FRCPA   Chapter 12
Head
Department of Chemical Pathology
St Vincent's Hospital, Sydney, Australia

D. J. Chisholm AO, MBBS, FRACP   Chapter 12
Professor and Head
Diabetes and Metabolism Research Program
Garvan Institute of Medical Research
St Vincent's Hospital, Sydney, Australia

J. R. Stockigt MD, FRACP, FRCPA
Professor of Medicine
Department of Endocrinology and Diabetes
Ewan Downie Metabolic Unit
Alfred Hospital, Prahan, Australia

Chapter 13

L. G. Olson MBBS, BSc, MLitt, PhD, FRACP
Senior Lecturer
Department of Medicine
John Hunter Hospital, Newcastle, Australia

Chapter 14

T. H. Mathew MBBS, FRACP
Associate Professor and Director
Renal Unit
The Queen Elizabeth Hospital, Woodville, Australia

Chapter 15

T. H. Mathew MBBS, FRACP
Associate Professor and Director
Renal Unit
The Queen Elizabeth Hospital, Woodville, Australia

Chapter 16

W. R. Pitney
Late Emeritus Professor
Department of Medicine
University of NSW, Sydney, Australia

Chapter 17

R. A. Dunstan PhD
School of Biomedical Sciences
Curtin University of Technology
Perth, Australia

Chapter 17

F. Firkin MBBS, BSc(Med), PhD, FRACP, FRCPA
Associate Professor, Department of Medicine
University of Melbourne
Director of Clinical Haematology
St Vincent's Hospital, Melbourne, Australia

Chapter 18

B. Rush MBBS, FRACP, FRCPA
Head
Department of Laboratory Haematology
St Vincent's Hospital, Melbourne, Australia

J. Metz MD, DSc(Med), FRCPath, FCAP,
DSc(Hon Causa)
Haematologist
Dorevitch Pathology
Fairfield, Australia

J. McPherson
Senior Lecturer in Medicine
Faculty of Medicine and Health Sciences
University of Newcastle, Newcastle, Australia

A. Street
Senior Staff Specialist in Haematology and Director
Haemophilia Centre
The Alfred Hospital, Melbourne, Australia

R. Baker MBBS, BMedSc, FRACP, FRCPA
Consultant Haematologist
Clinical Thrombosis Unit
Department of Haematology
Royal Perth Hospital, Perth, Australia

J. F. Mahony MBBS, FRACP
Clinical Associate Professor and Renal Physician
Department of Renal Medicine
Royal North Shore Hospital, Sydney, Australia

S. Nicholson BAppSci
Victorian Infectious Diseases Reference Laboratory,
Melbourne, Australia

I. Gust AO
Professor
Department of Microbiology and Immunology
University of Melbourne, Melbourne, Australia

D. Siebert Chapter 24
Director of Clinical Virology
Queensland Health Pathology Service
Royal Brisbane Hospital, Brisbane, Australia

S. A. Locarnini MBBS, BSc(Hons), PhD, FRC(Path) Chapter 24
Associate Professor
Victorian Infectious Diseases Reference Laboratory
Melbourne, Australia

A. M. Breschkin BA, PhD, MASM Chapter 25
Senior Scientist
Victorian Infectious Diseases Reference Laboratory
Melbourne, Australia

C. J. Birch BSc, MSc, PhD Chapter 25
Senior Scientist
Victorian HIV Reference Laboratory, VIDRL
Melbourne, Australia

M. G. Catton BSc(Hons) MB, ChB, FRCPA Chapter 25
Medical Director and Head
Victorian Infectious Diseases Reference Laboratory
Melbourne, Australia

D. Badov Chapter 26
Consultant Gastroenterologist
Department of Gastroenterology
Frankston Hospital, Melbourne, Australia

D. Siebert Chapter 27
Director of Clinical Virology
Queensland Health Pathology Service
Royal Brisbane Hospital, Brisbane, Australia

A. M. Breschkin BA, PhD, MASM Chapter 27
Senior Scientist
Victorian Infectious Diseases Reference Laboratory
Melbourne, Australia

D. S. Bowden BSc(Hons), PhD
Victorian Infectious Diseases Reference Laboratory
Melbourne, Australia

Chapter 27

S. A. Locarnini MBBS, BSc(Hons), PhD, FRC(Path)
Associate Professor
Victorian Infectious Diseases Reference Laboratory
Melbourne, Australia

Chapter 27

D. Barraclough MBBS, FRACP
Rheumatologist
Royal Melbourne Hospital, Melbourne, Australia

Chapter 28

D. Barraclough MBBS, FRACP
Rheumatologist
Royal Melbourne Hospital, Melbourne, Australia

Chapter 29

B. J. Nankivell
Department of Renal Medicine
Westmead Hospital, Sydney, Australia

Chapter 30

N. A. Buckley
Senior Consultant in Clinical Pharmacology and
Toxicology
Department of Clinical Pharmacology
Royal Adelaide Hospital, Adelaide, Australia

Chapter 31

Acknowledgments

The editor would like to thank the following people for their assistance in the work which led to the production of this book:

- each chapter's contributors who, despite their busy schedules, met the deadlines
- J. S. Dowden and staff from *Australian Prescriber* for their advice and encouragement
- Meiling Voon and staff from McGraw-Hill for their cheerful guidance
- Dawn Carthew for her good-humoured secretarial contribution to the project
- my wife, Jan, and our family for their support.

What to do about abnormal laboratory results

T. I. Robertson

A biochemical profile in a symptomless male patient of 50 years shows a modestly elevated serum uric acid. Anti-gout medication lowers the level but causes a generalised skin rash that lasts for 3 months. A patient 55 years old, in hospital with a myocardial infarct, is found on a routine blood count to have a haemoglobin level of 11.0 g/dL. The stained film suggests iron deficiency. Follow-up investigation uncovers a symptomless carcinoma of the caecum which is successfully removed. These two examples, each initiated by a routine test, show, on the one hand, an annoying disability resulting from treatment that was probably unnecessary and, on the other, successful conclusion to the pursuit of an apparently minor abnormality.

We live in a maze of biochemical profiles, screening tests and routine investigations, a lot of them uncalled for and some presented to us by our patients themselves. A new category has been created: the symptomless patient with an investigational abnormality. These people are at special risk. Some of them have incipient, developing or subclinical disease and some have no disease at all. But all will be affected by the medical advice they receive. Neglect of an apparent triviality may be lethal but yet a clearly abnormal result may, in the patient's total interest, be best set aside. The advent of routine screening procedures has produced fresh problems and responsibilities and has tended to complicate rather than simplify medical management.

When should an abnormal result be considered undebatably abnormal? When should it be acted upon? How vigorously should it be pursued? When should it be ignored? The magnitude of the problem can be reduced at source by discrimination in the investigations requested in the first place. The fewer tests ordered in isolation—that is, without proper integration with history, physical examination and general consideration of the clinical problem—the less difficult will be their interpretation. If a patient requires investigation of any type, he or she deserves the courtesy of proper history and examination first.

It is unrealistic to deny the ease, advantages and extra information provided by the automated blood count and multiple biochemical analysis. An investigation should, however, be mounted by way of a working diagnosis to be proved or disproved and the results of all tests viewed in that light. It should not be an undisciplined fishing expedition. If it is practical for only selective tests to be requested, to advance the working hypothesis, these only should be ordered. Secondary tests may be needed after analysis of the primary ones but this is still the preferred approach. The practitioner advances his or her capabilities by being careful, even parsimonious, with investigations and by understanding them and their limitations. This applies to all levels of clinical practice, not least in the teaching hospitals.

Nevertheless the problem of interpreting more or less isolated abnormal results will always remain. Some of the difficulties in relation to particular tests are addressed by experts in the articles that follow.

Abnormal laboratory results

C. G. Fraser

The finding of an unexpected 'abnormal' laboratory result is not uncommon, particularly with current approaches in diagnosis, case-finding and monitoring in which many different tests are requested simultaneously. However, before clinical action is taken, there are a number of logical reasons for the unexpected abnormal test result that should be considered.

Due to much international discussion and the wide dissemination of guidelines from the International Federation of Clinical Chemistry through the laboratory medicine community, the term 'reference range' is now widely used in preference to the term 'normal range'. This supposedly minimises the many semantic difficulties with the word 'normal' and should clearly suggest that, just because a result is outside the limits of the reference interval, it does not necessarily imply that the person is diseased. Moreover, most will know that the reference interval is simply a statistical concept that ensures that the limits encompass 95% of the reference population. Thus, by definition, 5% of the apparently healthy population will have values outside the reference limits— 2.5% will have high values and 2.5% will have low values. These individuals are not necessarily unhealthy—merely different from the bulk of the population. The unexpected laboratory result may well have arisen because the test has been done on one of these healthy, but simply rather different, individuals.

Reference values are affected by many factors. These include endogenous factors such as age and gender. They also include very many exogenous factors such as time of day, relationship of sampling to intake of food, exercise, posture, stress and immobilisation. Laboratories often do examine the effects of some of these factors on their reference values and, provided that the test requestor gives correct information, particularly about age and sex, modern laboratory information systems will insert the appropriately stratified reference values on the test report, irrespective of whether paper or electronic. It is vital to note that reference values may be highly dependent on the analytical method that the laboratory uses, particularly for enzymes and hormones. Moreover, some reference values, such as glucose, depend on the type of sample—capillary blood is not the same as venous plasma. An unexplained abnormal laboratory result may arise because an inappropriate reference interval is used for comparison. Because reference values depend on population, laboratory methodology and workflow approaches, it is good practice to use only the values provided by the laboratory that performed the test. It is totally inappropriate to use reference values found in texts, books, diaries and the like. Undoubtedly, dependence on such sources will give rise to unexpected abnormal laboratory results.

Purely on statistical grounds, the more tests that are done, the higher the chance of finding an unexpected abnormal result. If one test is done, then 5% of the population lie outside the reference limits. If two unrelated tests are done, over 9% of the population lie outside the reference limits. When 20 tests are performed on the one patient, there will be as high as a 60% chance of observing at least one abnormal result.

Sometimes the unexpected abnormal laboratory result is said to be a 'laboratory error'. These are actually now rare. Modern analytical equipment generally uses the primary specimen tube used to collect the blood so that mix-up is uncommon. Laboratories have comprehensive internal quality control programs that monitor all facets of performance. They also participate in regional, national and international external quality assessment schemes, which allows inter-laboratory comparisons of performance. In many countries, laboratories have extensive accreditation procedures and compliance with all the standards is mandatory. However, it is admitted that unexpected laboratory results caused by error do still occur. Commonly, these are caused by mistakes made before the laboratory receives the specimen—for example, through patient misidentification at test request level, contamination of the sample by anticoagulants or IV fluids, prolonged venous stasis, and inadequate preservation or storage prior to the transportation of the specimen to the laboratory.

Although analytical methodology continues to improve with time, certain test procedures are not totally specific for the test they purport to measure. A number of commonly prescribed drugs do cross-react in current methods. The unexpected abnormal laboratory result may be due to such drug interference.

Laboratories report test results as single numbers. However, this number is a representation of a range of values, the width of which depends on inherent within-subject biological variation and on analytical imprecision. Every analytical method has some imprecision and this may be quite large for difficult-to-measure components, particularly those present in only very small amounts in body fluids. Thus, when a single numerical value is reported as being outside the reference interval, the range of readings that the single value actually means may, at least in part, overlap the reference interval. This is particularly so in borderline situations.

The natural history of many diseases is not fully understood as yet and it may be difficult to decide on the clinical implications of an unexpected abnormal result when no disease is apparent. Some would suggest that abnormal results are a sign of unsuspected disease. There is little objective evidence to support such a conclusion. A number of studies have examined the frequency with which unexpected laboratory results are found, particularly when the idea of performing a profile of common tests was in vogue. These studies have shown that, in general, the reasons for the unexpected abnormal laboratory results are far from clear.

Since there are many reasons for the unexpected abnormal result, the recommended approach is to seek the advice of the laboratory. Laboratory staff can assess whether the appropriate reference values were used and give advice on the many factors that influence such values—these are very fully documented in the literature of laboratory medicine. Moreover, laboratory staff can quickly check on the possibility of error since most laboratories retain all specimens for some time and can often track the location using computer systems. In addition, the possibility of an in vivo or in vitro drug test interaction can be assessed—again these are very fully documented in the literature of laboratory medicine. Laboratory staff will have knowledge of biological and analytical sources of variation and will be able to advise on the probability that the unexpected abnormal laboratory result does lie within the reference interval. Laboratory staff may be able to advise on the likelihood that pathological processes or latent disease is present and may well be able to suggest the most appropriate further investigations to clarify the situation.

Unexpected abnormal laboratory results are a common finding. If there are no logical clinical reasons for the unexpected, a carefully collected repeat specimen should always be submitted for analysis before other laboratory tests are requested or clinical action initiated.

What does the reference range of a biochemical screen test mean?

G. M. Kellerman

The concept of normal individual is one of the most difficult to define in clinical medicine. A working definition such as an individual who has no detectable disease and no demonstrable excess tendency to develop diseases relevant to the situation under discussion has the benefit of leaving the uncertainty of undiagnosed disease in the definition, as well as permitting risk factor analysis at an appropriate level. But does such a normal individual have a normal value for a particular biochemical test? Normal individuals vary in many respects—age, sex, genetic make-up, lifestyle, preferred diet, exercise—and their values for a given test also vary, generating a range of normal values. A few of these apparently normal individuals have as yet undiagnosed disease and, more importantly, others may be in a group as yet unrecognised due to lack of appropriate research, with an increased risk factor for a particular disease to develop in, say, 20 years time. These latter will surely be excluded when research has documented the risk factor— consider how the concepts of borderline hypertension, prediabetes or atherosclerosis have developed over the years.

The normal range for a particular test can be analysed statistically as described in standard textbooks.[1,2] If we assume a Gaussian distribution, simple prediction is possible of the proportion who will fall within so many standard deviations of the mean. Other types of distribution can be manipulated by special statistical methods. For many (but not all) tests, a given individual has a far narrower variation during health than does the population as a whole and an accurate knowledge of their personal normal range could be of value in assessing their state of health. Without such information, we can use only the broader population-based normal range in our assessment of the patient, and our decision depends on where the person's own normal value happened to be and how far the value has moved with the disease process. There is uncertainty in decision making even if we have a previous normal value for the particular person. Furthermore, no analytical technique is perfect: there is always some error, leading either to non-reproducibility of a result on the same specimen (lack of precision) or an incorrect, but reproducible, answer (lack of accuracy). Clinical laboratories strive to minimise these errors with extensive and expensive quality control systems, and thus to increase the predictive value of their results.

Clinical biochemists have accepted for some years the position described above, and now define not a *normal* but a *reference range*. Values within the reference range do not exclude disease affecting the parameter under examination, but do not raise suspicion of its presence. Values outside the reference range are a signal that thought is necessary—and the further away the results from the reference range, the more likely is the presence of a disease process. If the reference range is set too narrow, too high a proportion of normal people will have suspicion cast on them (false positive results or low *specificity*); if the reference range is set too broad, too many abnormal individuals will be missed (false negative results or low *sensitivity*). A compromise is always necessary in such circumstances between specificity and sensitivity, the exact decision depending on the prevalence of the disease in the population being studied.[3, 4] In most hospital laboratories it is customary to set the reference range to include the central 95% of values of people presumed normal. Such a procedure yields only an index of suspicion—it is wrong to treat one in 20 of the population for a hypothetical condition by a treatment appropriate to a real condition; *doctors should treat patients with problems, not analytical results.*

Experienced clinicians, therefore, develop an index of increasing suspicion, combining the degree of deviation of a particular value from its reference range with results of other tests, observations of the patient and so on. They are really combining a number of probabilities, gained from their experience, appropriate for the community in which they work. They realise that a value within the reference range also has a given probability of being compatible with disease—less than for those outside the range but still not zero—and skilful manipulation of probabilities often can help in deciding between two possible diagnoses.[5] They avoid the trap that the more unrelated tests that are done on the one patient, the greater the chance that one or more will fall outside the reference range. They use their clinical judgement to avoid overreaction, with further tests and investigations galore—the familiar investigation and treatment of the asterisks and not of the patient. Such clinicians can often combine results of several tests to add to their predictive accuracy (e.g. reciprocal movements of calcium and phosphate and appropriate changes in alkaline phosphatase) and research suggests that the combination of test results (even within the reference range) by sophisticated techniques such as discriminant function analysis may help to identify the probability of a given hypothesis. However, such analysis has proven to be very population-dependent, so that even in neighbouring parts of a city, coefficients may prove to be non-transferable, thus limiting the value of this method.

One final warning: how does a laboratory establish its reference range? Where do the normal subjects come from? Are the results from young, healthy, fit male football players (or doctors, nurses, blood donors, school children, volunteers, army conscripts) applicable to the inhabitants of old age homes, pregnant women or newborn babies? Where a risk factor for a given result has been proposed (e.g. cholesterol and ischaemic heart disease), where does one draw the line of normality to establish the reference range? Can we use a hospital population, recognise that most results are normal and just throw away those from the obviously diseased? Current practice tends to either accept this last alternative as one way, or to collect a suitable set of apparently normal persons (age-matched, sex-matched etc., if appropriate), with statistical manipulations. However, we must not forget that this approach contains an element of personal value judgement, which may change in the future as methodology and knowledge improve. Long may it remain so, for our current use of laboratory test results is neither precise nor accurate, even if the tests themselves are. There is no substitute for thought, experience and research.

REFERENCES

1 Kringle R. O. and Bogovich M. Statistical procedures. In: Tietz, *Textbook of Clinical Chemistry*. 3rd edn. Philadelphia: WB Saunders, 1999, pp. 265–309.

2 Feinstein A. R. *Clinical Biostatistics*. St Louis: Mosby, 1977.

3 Henry R. J. and Reed A. H. Normal values and the use of laboratory results for the detection of disease. In: Henry R. J. and Reed A. H., eds. *Clinical Chemistry*, Principles and Techniques. Hagerstown: Harper and Row, 1974, pp. 343–71.

4 Watson R. A. and Tang D. B. The predictive value of prostatic acid phosphatase as a screening test for prostatic cancer. *N Engl J Med* 1980; 303: 497–9.

5 Gorry G. A., Pauker S. G. and Schwartz W. B. The diagnostic importance of the normal finding. *N Engl J Med* 1978; 298: 486–9.

Plasma creatinine

4

T. H. Mathew

SYNOPSIS

The plasma creatinine concentration is the single most useful clinical measure of renal function. It is easy to measure, varies little throughout the day and can be converted to a measurement of glomerular filtration rate with reasonable accuracy by the application of a simple formula. For the clinician to use the plasma creatinine appropriately it is necessary to understand its relationship to the glomerular filtration rate and the impact of the clinical variables on creatinine production.

Introduction

The plasma creatinine concentration is useful as a clinical test of renal function (glomerular filtration rate) because the daily production rate is constant within 10% (unlike urea production which is influenced by dietary protein intake, drugs, gastrointestinal bleeding and mild dehydration) and the excretion of creatinine is mainly renal. The only other clinically useful way of determining the glomerular filtration rate is the creatinine clearance test. This requires a prolonged timed collection of urine (usually 24 hours) as shorter collection periods tend to give less accurate results. The inherent difficulties in accomplishing complete collections of urine have led to this test being used only rarely. It is useful to document glomerular filtration rate at the beginning of a patient's course of management but too demanding to use for regular monitoring of renal function.

In general terms changes in the plasma creatinine parallel changes in glomerular filtration rate and are therefore indicative of the overall stability or otherwise of progressive renal conditions. A change concentration of 30 µmol/L or more is regarded as clinically significant.

Technical aspects

Plasma creatinine is usually assayed on an autoanalyser by the colorimetric-dependent alkaline picrate method. It is usually accurate to within 10–20 µmol/L. The assay can be significantly interfered with (increased by 50–150 µmol/L) by acetoacetate in diabetic ketoacidosis or the presence of cefoxitin or flucytosine. In most clinical situations the plasma creatinine concentration is reliable and varies less than 10% from day to day in a steady state. It must be remembered that in a non-steady-state plasma creatinine should not be used to determine glomerular filtration rate.

Physiological aspects

Creatinine is excreted almost entirely by the kidney except in severe renal failure when 5–10% finds its way into the bowel. In the kidney, creatinine is freely filtered. About 15% of the final urinary creatinine comes from secretion of creatinine (an organic cation in the physiological pH range) through the organic cation pathway. This secretion makes it susceptible to competitive inhibition by other cations including drugs and their metabolites. Trimethoprim and cimetidine are two commonly used agents that interfere with the secretory pathway and may cause a self-limited and reversible rise in plasma creatinine of 30–40 µmol/L. Cimetidine has been recommended for routine use during the collection of a creatinine clearance in order to improve the accuracy of the calculated creatinine clearance in measuring a true glomerular filtration rate by removing the tubular component.

The production of creatinine relates closely to total muscle mass. In small patients (usually female) whose muscle mass is reduced in relation to body surface area, the production rate is relatively less and abnormally low plasma creatinine concentrations (35–50 µmol/L) may be seen. These low concentrations are also seen early in normal pregnancy where the glomerular filtration rate is increased by 35–50%.

When the filtering surface of the glomerulus (effectively the same as the number of functioning nephrons) is reduced in area through progressive disease the plasma creatinine will rise. This inverse relationship is not linear but in mathematical terms is that of a hyperbolic parabola (Fig. 4.1). In simple terms, this relationship means that, whatever the level considered, as the number of nephrons halves, the plasma creatinine concentration will double. For example, a rise in the plasma creatinine from 80 to 160 µmol/L represents the same fractional change (50%) as a rise from 500 to 1000 µmol/L. In terms of absolute numbers of nephrons lost, the smaller rise in plasma creatinine represents a much greater loss.

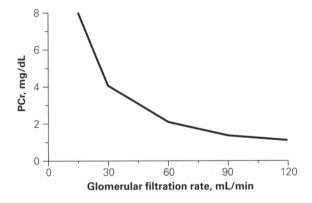

FIGURE 4.1 Plasma creatinine and GFR

Idealised steady-state relationship between the plasma creatinine concentration (PCr) and the GFR. A fall in GFR decreases creatinine filtration and produces a proportionate rise in the plasma creatinine concentration.

The normal range of plasma creatinine is 50–120 µmol/L. The distribution of plasma creatinine in males and females is shown in Figure 4.2. If in a particular patient a plasma creatinine of 50 µmol/L is shown to equate with a normal glomerular filtration rate of

120 mL/min, reduction of the nephron numbers by 50% (e.g. by donor nephrectomy) will result in a glomerular filtration rate of 60 mL/min and a rise in the plasma creatinine to 100 µmol/L—still well within the 'normal' range. This exemplifies the difficulty of interpreting plasma creatinine concentrations when the result is in the high normal range. In clinical practice, this idealised example is confounded by the fact that both some hypertrophy of residual nephrons and some increase in tubular secretion (seen only until this mechanism is saturated when the plasma creatinine reaches about 150 µmol/L) occur. These two factors contribute to a lower than might be expected plasma creatinine concentration.

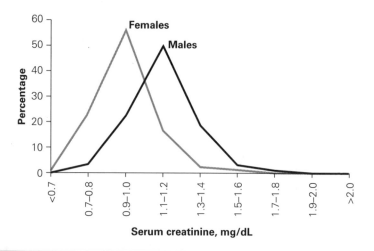

FIGURE 4.2 Distribution of serum creatinine

Distribution of the serum creatinine (in mg/dL) among United States males and females for the years 1988 to 1994 (12 years or older in age). Multiply values by 88.4 to convert to units of mmol/L. (Data from Jones C. A., et al. Serum creatinine levels in the US population: third National Health and Nutrition Examination Survey. *Am J Kidney Dis* 1998; 6: 992–9.)

The effect of age is also important. Several studies using creatinine clearance to measure glomerular filtration rate have suggested that there is a loss of glomerular filtration rate with increasing years of about 0.75 mL/min/year beyond the age of 40 years. However the production rate of creatinine falls as muscle mass reduces in old age and this makes creatinine clearance a poor technique to use for this purpose. A study using insulin clearance to determine glomerular filtration rate found the majority of patients not in heart failure (mean age 69 years) to have clearances above 100 mL/min. Thus the dogma of age being associated with an inexorable decline in renal function is being challenged. In the presence of disease (e.g. heart failure) renal function does decline but healthy old age is not invariably associated with a reduced glomerular filtration rate.

Is the result abnormal?

In an individual in whom the plasma creatinine is marginally raised, it may be impossible to decide whether the result is abnormal without performing additional tests. A single plasma creatinine concentration that is considered abnormal should always be repeated, preferably in the fasting state. A recently ingested large meal of meat can raise the plasma creatinine by 50 μmol/L (since muscle contains creatinine). If the marginally raised plasma creatinine concentration is confirmed, the next test should be the determination of the glomerular filtration rate by a 24-hour creatinine clearance or isotope technique. A plasma creatinine concentration higher than 140 μmol/L should always be regarded as abnormal and further investigated.

What action is needed if the plasma creatinine concentration is abnormal?

An abnormal result should be pursued actively until an explanation is found. There will often be an indication of the cause of the abnormality by the bedside. The first and simplest cause to exclude is mild dehydration which may be significant yet subtle, particularly in the elderly patient. If dehydration is suspected, elevation of the body weight by 1–2 kg through increased salt and water intake will clarify the situation. In the absence of dehydration or other causes of reduced blood volume, the drug history should be considered. Reversible renal function impairment may occur with diuretics, antihypertensives (particularly angiotensin-active agents), and with all the non-steroidal anti-inflammatory agents (including the cox-2 selective inhibitors). When these agents are combined (the so-called double or triple whammy effect), the risk of renal function impairment escalates and such impairment is a common cause of a raised plasma creatinine, especially in the elderly.

In the absence of drugs or dehydration, a detailed history and examination may point to the cause. A positive family history may indicate polycystic kidney disease or familial nephritis. A history of oedema or dark urine suggests glomerulonephritis, a history of childhood enuresis and later urinary infections suggests reflux nephropathy, and one of loin pain with dysuria raises the possibility of analgesic nephropathy.

The next investigation should be urinalysis and culture of a freshly voided midstream specimen, with quantitative cell counting, determination of red cell morphology under phase contrast microscopy, and a careful search for casts. If evidence of nephritis is found (glomerular red cells and casts with proteinuria), referral for consideration of renal biopsy is recommended. If proteinuria alone is found, the 24-hour urine protein excretion should de determined (creatinine clearance can be performed on the same specimen). Even with small amounts of urinary protein (0.3–1.0 g/24 hours), renal biopsy should be considered in the presence of impaired renal function. If there is evidence of infection in the urine (polymorphs and organisms on microscopy or a positive culture), the next step should be to determine the renal anatomy by renal imaging (ultrasound +/– CT spiral urography). Obstruction will be evident at this stage. If the urine is normal (negative for cells, protein and organisms) and the imaging normal, then it is still necessary to investigate if there is evidence of a definite abnormality of renal function. In this rare situation one should proceed to renal angiography to exclude a vascular cause, and renal biopsy that will diagnose an interstitial cause such as medullary cystic disease or interstitial nephritis.

Summary

The plasma creatinine is the major clinical tool available day to day for the estimation of renal excretory function. It is subject to few extrarenal variables and, when a steady renal state exists and the plasma creatinine is adjusted for body size, it may be converted to a clinically useful and reasonably accurate estimation of glomerular filtration rate. It is essential, for the plasma creatinine to be used effectively, to have a full understanding of the relationship between plasma creatinine and glomerular filtration rate.

Serum potassium

5

G. S. Stokes and E. P. MacCarthy

Introduction

Hypokalaemia and hyperkalaemia are potentially lethal disorders, often iatrogenic, which can be handled readily once the underlying mechanism is identified. A finding of low serum potassium concentration (<3.5 mmol/L) or high serum potassium concentration (>5.5 mmol/L) is an indication for urgent notification of the responsible doctor.

Technical aspects

As red blood cells are rich in potassium, high levels can result from stasis or haemolysis in vitro, or from prolonged tourniquet application.

Is the result abnormal?

Before any definitive action is taken, it should be confirmed that the result, particularly in the case of hyperkalaemia, genuinely reflects the prevailing plasma potassium levels. A repeat sample should be obtained without a tourniquet and centrifuged promptly. Immediate evidence of dangerously abnormal levels may be found in an electrocardiograph. Some causes of abnormal potassium levels are shown in Table 5.1.

TABLE 5.1 Some causes of abnormal potassium levels

CAUSES OF HYPOKALAEMIA	CAUSES OF HYPERKALAEMIA
GASTROINTESTINAL Vomiting, gastric suction Diarrhoea, purgative abuse	METABOLIC AND RENAL Acidosis Renal failure Hypoaldosteronism Addison's disease

METABOLIC AND RENAL
Renal tubular acidosis
   Liddle's syndrome
Primary aldosteronism
   (Conn's syndrome)
Secondary aldosteronism
   (oedematous states,
   Bartter's syndrome,
   Gitelman's syndrome,
   hypertension)
Glucocorticoid excess (Cushing's
   disease, ectopic ACTH,
   exogenous steroids)
Alkalosis
	TISSUE DAMAGE
	Burns, massive trauma
	Haemolysis
	
	DRUGS
	Spironolactone
	Amiloride
	Triamterene
	Potassium supplements
	   (excess or lack)
	ACE inhibitors
	Angiotensin II receptor
	   antagonists
	Digitalis (excess)
	Suxamethonium

DRUGS Carbenoxolone, liquorice Diuretics Insulin (excess) Corticosteroids	

Is the abnormality iatrogenic?

In explaining abnormal serum potassium levels, costly investigation can often be avoided by early recognition of the role of drugs. Thiazide diuretics probably constitute the most common cause of mild hypokalaemia, although it should be emphasised that most patients receiving these agents in conventional dosage, with or without potassium supplements, never become hypokalaemic. Chlorthalidone in high doses is more likely than the thiazides to produce hypokalaemia, and indapamide rather less. When frusemide is used to treat the anxious obese (a dubious indication) or women with 'cyclic oedema', the dosage may be increased surreptitiously, inducing potassium depletion. Potassium depletion is more prevalent, too, in patients treated with diuretics for chronic oedematous states. Patients on such treatment require regular measurement of their serum potassium. A large intake of liquorice can also lower serum potassium levels.[1]

Laxative abuse is another common cause of unexpected hypokalaemia. Whereas the patient with infective or inflammatory bowel disease severe enough to cause potassium depletion will be symptomatic, the individual with a bowel fixation may regard his explosive, liquid motions as appropriate.

Although its causes are fewer than those of hypokalaemia, hyperkalaemia is of more immediate danger to the patient, with a high risk of a dangerous and possibly fatal outcome.

Hyperkalaemia can be precipitated by the use of potassium-sparing diuretics, such as amiloride, triamterene or spironolactone, in patients with chronic renal failure or those taking concurrent potassium supplements. Hyperkalaemia can also occur in patients taking drugs which inhibit the renin-angiotensin system, such as angiotensin converting enzyme (ACE) inhibitors or angiotensin II receptor antagonists. There have been reports, too, of hyperkalaemia occurring in patients with renal disease given indomethacin or beta adrenergic blocking drugs.[2, 3]

Hyperkalaemia will be provoked more readily in elderly or diabetic patients with hyporeninaemic hypoaldosteronism.

What action is needed if result is abnormal?
What action should be taken if hyperkalaemia is found?

Whatever the history may reveal in the way of suspect drugs, hyperkalaemia should be regarded as possibly indicative of renal impairment which should be sought carefully. In a state of stable renal impairment, hyperkalaemia can usually be controlled by correction of acidosis (using oral sodium bicarbonate provided the patient is not oliguric or fluid-overloaded) and reduction of foods rich in potassium, together with the elimination of any precipitating factors such as dehydration or renal tract obstruction or infection. The presence of acidosis indicates severe renal failure and a patient presenting in this state requires thorough investigation and aggressive treatment. If renal function is normal, investigations should be carried out to eliminate adrenal insufficiency as the cause of hyperkalaemia.

In cases of hypokalaemia, how can the route of potassium loss be definitely established?

If the history and physical examination have failed to identify it clearly, it is simple to establish whether the route of potassium loss is gastrointestinal or renal. The key test is to measure serum potassium concentration in relation to the concurrent 24-hour urinary excretion of potassium.[4] If the patient has been taking diuretics or potassium supplements, these are suspended 5 days before the test. In patients with extrarenal potassium loss, urinary potassium excretion will be appropriately low in compensation (less than 30 mmol/24 hours) while hypokalaemia from renal tubular disease or adrenocortical overactivity or surreptitious diuretic or liquorice ingestion will be accompanied by a urinary potassium excretion inappropriately high for the low plasma level (over 30 mmol/24 hours for a plasma potassium of 3.5 mmol/hour or less).

A further simple test which can support a diagnosis of surreptitious laxative abuse is titration of the urine with alkali to a pH of 10: appearance of a pink colouration in the urine at a pH between 8 and 10 suggests the presence of phenolphthalein, a common constituent of laxative preparations. Inspection of the colonic mucosa by sigmoidoscopy may reveal melanosis coli, in which there is black pigmentation due to chronic laxative abuse.

While not posing such an urgent problem as hyperkalaemia, uncorrected hypokalaemia may lead to muscle weakness and, occasionally, cardiac or respiratory arrest. It should be particularly remembered that, in cardiac failure, diuretics may induce hypokalaemia which dangerously sensitises the heart to digoxin.

Summary

The first thing to think of with abnormal serum potassium concentration is whether it is drug-induced. Systemic causes to consider are tissue trauma, gastrointestinal losses, renal failure and adrenal insufficiency.

REFERENCES

1 Conn J. W., Rovner D. R. and Cohen E. L. Liquorice-induced pseudoaldosteronism. Hypertension, hypokalemia, aldosteronopenia,

Abnormal laboratory results

and suppressed plasma renin activity. *JAMA* 1968; 205: 492–6.

2 Tan S. Y., Shapiro R., Franco R., et al. Indomethacin induced prostaglandin inhibition with hyperkalemia: reversible cause of hyporeninemic hypoaldosteronism. *Clin Res* 1977; 25: 598A.

3 Pederson E. B. and Kornerup H. J. Relationship between plasma aldosterone concentration and plasma potassium in patients with essential hypertension during alprenolol treatment. *Acta Med Scand* 1976; 200: 263–7.

4 Kaplan N. M. Hypokalaemia in the hypertensive patient, with observations on the incidence of primary aldosteronism. *Ann Intern Med* 1967; 66: 1079–90.

6 | Calcium

R. G. Larkins

Introduction

The approach to an abnormal plasma calcium result differs according to whether the plasma calcium was measured because of specific symptoms or signs, or whether the abnormal result was as an incidental finding, e.g. during multiphasic screening.

This chapter will be confined to a consideration of the incidental detection of an abnormal plasma calcium.

Is the result abnormal?

Apart from the possibility of laboratory error, falsely elevated values can be due to haemoconcentration associated with the use of a tourniquet. In addition, in patients with abnormal plasma protein concentrations, appropriate corrections should be made.[1] Marginal abnormalities should be confirmed by repeated tests.

The quoted 'normal range' is calculated in most laboratories to include 95% of normal individuals, so even a confirmed and corrected value slightly outside the normal range need not indicate disease.

Direct measurement of ionised, dialysable or ultrafiltrable calcium avoids problems associated with protein-binding, and is being used more frequently.

Causes and effects of hypercalcaemia

The major causes of hypercalcaemia are listed in Table 6.1. In hospital practice, malignancy is the most common cause,[2] but in asymptomatic patients, primary hyperparathyroidism is much more frequent. Clinical assessment should be directed particularly towards eliciting (1) symptoms of hypercalcaemia and its consequences such as thirst, polyuria, constipation, renal colic; and (2) symptoms and signs of the cause of hypercalcaemia. Particular attention should be paid to ingestion of thiazides and antacids containing calcium and sodium bicarbonate, and to symptoms suggestive of malignancy. A lack of evidence of other causes of hypercalcaemia suggests hyperparathyroidism.

TABLE 6.1 Some causes of hypercalcaemia

1 Primary hyperparathyroidism
2 Malignant disease
   (a) with bone involvement, e.g. metastatic carcinoma of the breast
   (b) without bone involvement, e.g. squamous cell carcinoma of the lung, carcinoma of the kidney
   (c) haematological malignancy, e.g. multiple myeloma, lymphoma
3 Sarcoidosis
4 Vitamin D intoxication
5 Milk alkali syndrome
6 Immobilisation
7 Thyrotoxicosis
8 Thiazide diuretics
9 Familial hypocalciuric hypercalcaemia

A positive family history of hypercalcaemia raises the possibility of multiple endocrine neoplasia with hyperparathyroidism and of familial hypocalciuric hypercalcaemia. Both these conditions are transmitted as Mendelian-dominant characteristics.

What further tests are required?

The diagnosis of hyperparathyroidism is supported by a low plasma phosphate, a raised plasma chloride and a low-normal plasma bicarbonate. Raised plasma parathyroid hormone provides strong evidence for the diagnosis if renal function is normal. X-rays of the hands may reveal the characteristic subperiosteal erosions of hyperparathyroidism, and other skeletal X-rays may reveal bone cysts in hyperparathyroidism or evidence of metastases in malignant hypercalcaemia. Bone scan may reveal metastases. X-ray of the abdomen may reveal renal or ureteric calculi or nephrocalcinosis in patients with hyperparathyroidism or sarcoidosis, and an intravenous pyelogram may be indicated to exclude carcinoma of the kidney if microscopic haematuria is present.

Serum angiotensin-converting enzyme (ACE) levels are raised in patients with hypercalcaemia due to sarcoidosis. Serum 25 OH vitamin D levels are elevated in patients with vitamin D intoxication. Plasma PTH-P is elevated in many patients with malignant hypercalcaemia.[3]

Management

Patients with serum calcium values of 3 mmol/L or less do not usually require urgent treatment. If a cause of hypercalcaemia apart from primary hyperparathyroidism is found, this is treated on its merits. There is controversy concerning the correct management of asymptomatic patients with presumptive primary hyperparathyroidism.[4] While the condition may be associated with progressive bone loss[5] and the risk of renal impairment, renal calculi, hypercalcaemic crises, peptic ulcers and pancreatitis, in most patients the condition follows a benign course.[5, 6, 7] In elderly patients, without specific indications for surgical intervention such as renal calculi, renal impairment, bone disease, pancreatitis, peptic ulceration or severe hypercalcaemia (greater than 2.85 mmol/L) observation is a reasonable approach.[8] In patients where neck exploration is decided upon, an experienced surgeon is usually able to find and correct the parathyroid abnormality. Intravenous pamidronate treatment has simplified the management of malignant hypercalcaemia. Ultrasound or isotope scanning may be helpful in preoperative localisation of the adenoma. (See Fig. 6.1.)

Causes and effects of hypocalcaemia

The main causes of hypocalcaemia are shown in Table 6.2. Postsurgical hypoparathyroidism is the most common cause in asymptomatic adults. In younger patients, idiopathic hypoparathyroidism (probably autoimmune in origin) is the most common cause, and it may be associated with other autoimmune endocrine deficiency diseases, and with mucocutaneous candidiasis.

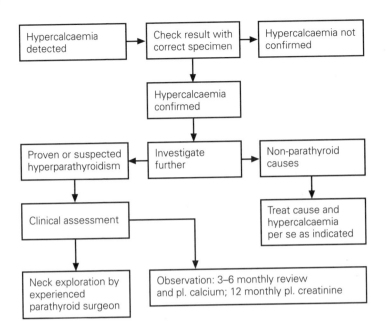

FIGURE 6.1 Hypercalcaemia—management

TABLE 6.2 Some causes of hypocalcaemia

1 Hypoparathyroidism: idiopathic
                                 post-surgical
                                 pseudo
2 Malabsorptive and nutritional vitamin D deficiency
  (osteomalacia and rickets)
3 Chronic renal disease
4 Hypomagnesaemia

    Vitamin D deficiency, commonly associated with malabsorption, may present with hypocalcaemia at any age, although osteomalacia or rickets can also occur with a normal plasma calcium.

    Symptoms and signs of hypocalcaemia should be sought. They include paraesthesiae and carpal or pedal spasm, nail changes, cataracts and epilepsy. It may be possible to provoke carpal spasm by inflating the blood pressure cuff to greater than systolic pressure (Trousseau's sign), and a facial twitch may be elicited by tapping over the facial nerve (Chvostek's sign).

A history of thyroidectomy or a neck scar may be present, and symptoms and signs of renal impairment and malabsorption should be sought. A family history of hypocalcaemia may be present in pseudohypoparathyroidism which may be diagnosed by the characteristic skeletal features.

What further tests are required?

Plasma phosphate tends to be high in hypoparathyroidism and chronic renal failure, and low in nutritional and malabsorptive osteomalacia and rickets. Skeletal alkaline phosphatase is usually raised in osteomalacia or rickets and renal failure. Plasma parathyroid hormone is undetectable or inappropriately low in hypoparathyroidism, but raised in hypocalcaemia due to chronic renal failure, osteomalacia, rickets and pseudohypoparathyroidism. Renal function should be checked and malabsorption excluded. Plasma 25-hydroxyvitamin D (25-OH-D) levels are very low in patients with hypocalcaemia associated with malabsorption or nutritional osteomalacia or rickets, and skeletal survey may show osteopenia and possibly pseudofractures.

Management

Even if asymptomatic, hypocalcaemia associated with hypoparathyroidism or pseudohypoparathyroidism probably justifies treatment with calcitriol and oral calcium because of the risks of cataracts and epilepsy if left untreated. The treatment must be monitored carefully with plasma calcium determination at least 3 monthly to avoid hypercalcaemia. (See Fig. 6.2.)

In patients with hypocalcaemia associated with osteomalacia or rickets due to malabsorption or nutritional causes, the most appropriate form of vitamin D replacement to use is ergocalciferol, as there is a wide margin between therapeutic and toxic doses in these conditions.

Summary

Routine screening leads to abnormal plasma calcium results in about 5% of the community.[8] The abnormality may represent a laboratory error, an extreme of a normal distribution, a benign condition which from the subject's point of view would have been better undetected, a significant but untreatable underlying disease

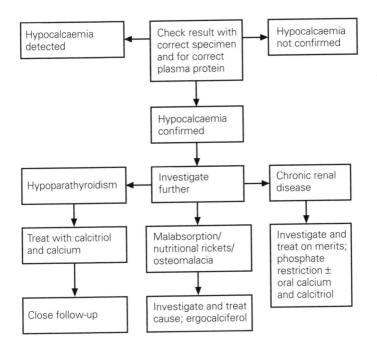

FIGURE 6.2 Hypocalcaemia—management

or a significant and treatable disorder. The relatively benign natural history of primary hyperparathyroidism makes it likely that only a small percentage of cases fall into the last category. The extent and direction of investigation and the final management decided upon should be based on the individual situation, but enthusiasm to get to the bottom of the problem and to obtain biochemical normalisation should be tempered by remembering constantly that the subject did not present complaining of the calcium abnormality, and in most cases it is not certain that it will do them any harm.

REFERENCES

1 Parfitt A. M. Investigation of disorders of the parathyroid glands. *Clin Endocrinol Metab* 1974; 3: 451–74.

2   Aitken R. E., Bartley P. C., Bryant S. J. and Lloyd H. M. The effect of multiphasic biochemical screening on the diagnosis of primary hyperparathyroidism. *Aust NZ J Med* 1975; 5: 224–6.

3   Wysolmerski J. J. and Broachis A. C. Hypercalcaemia of malignancy: the central role of parathyroid hormone-related protein. *Annu Rev Med* 1994; 45: 189–200.

4   Utiger R. D. Treatment of primary hyperparathyroidism. *N Engl J Med* 1999; 341: 1301–2.

5   Kaplan R. A., Snyder W. I. I., Stewart A. and Pak C. Y. Metabolic effects of parathyroidectomy in asymptomatic primary hyperparathyroidism. *J Clin Endocrinol Metab* 1976; 42: 415–26.

6   Rubinoff H., McCarthy N. and Hiatt R.A. Hypercalcemia: long-term follow-up with matched controls. *J Chronic Dis* 1983; 36: 859–68.

7   Posen S., Clifton-Bligh P., Reeve T. S., Wagstaffe C. and Wilkinson M. Is parathyroidectomy of benefit in primary hyperparathyroidism? *Q J Med* 1985; 54: 241–51.

8   Potts J. T., ed. Proceedings of the NIH consensus development conference on diagnosis and management of asymptomatic primary hyperparathyroidism. *J Bone Miner Res* 1991; 6(52): 9–13.

Managing hyperlipidaemia: criteria for investigating

7

P. Nestel

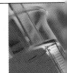

Key principles

Major clinical trials reported in the last decade have established new principles.

Lipid risk factors

The key conclusion from the three major secondary intervention trials (4S, LIPID, CARE) is that the reduction in clinical coronary heart disease events (mortality, recurrent infarction etc.) is proportional to low density lipoprotein (LDL) lowering even when initial levels are normal. Similar findings emerge from the two primary prevention trials (WOSCOPS, AFCAPS). Lowering triglyceride and raising high density lipoprotein (HDL) cholesterol (VA-HIT) has recently also been shown to reduce CHD events. The latter trial, in which LDL levels were normal, shows, together with much epidemiological data, that triglycerides are an independent risk factor and further increase the risk in combination with low HDL or high LDL. Reductions of 25–30% in LDL cholesterol have resulted in lowering first or further events by 30–35%.

Concept of total risk

Full assessment and management of dyslipidaemia (abnormal plasma lipids) requires *full evaluation of other risk factors*. If raised cholesterol is an isolated factor then treatment should not be as vigorous as in those with multiple factors, especially if coronary heart disease (CHD) is present.

Evaluating total or absolute risk for elevated LDL

The following multiples are approximations:
- Existing CHD: five times the risk
- Diabetes: four times the risk in women, less in men
- Hypertension and associated left-ventricular pathology—each doubles the risk
- Family history of CHD under the age of 65 doubles the risk
- Smoking doubles the risk
- Low HDL cholesterol, *itself a powerful independent risk factor*, doubles the risk
- Other lifestyle factors (obesity, physical inactivity) and new factors such as homocysteinaemia raise the risk by less certain multiples. *Charts of absolute or total risk are available from health organisations, pharmaceutical companies and the Internet, and are valuable in assessing the need for drugs and in motivating patients.*

Critical importance of CHD

Identifying such patients and treating them strenuously, even when plasma lipids appear normal, *represents the most cost-effective strategy for reducing further events.*

Target for LDL-lowering

Trials show that for high-risk patients and *in those with existing CHD, the target is <3 mmol/L.* Further trials are in progress to determine the extent of benefit from lowering LDL further. There are targets also for triglycerides and for HDL cholesterol but these have not been substantiated in sufficient clinical trials.

Benefits for most population groups

Recent trials have established benefit for menopausal women that is as great as for men and for the elderly at least into their 70s. Given the powerful effect of age on CHD incidence, lipid-lowering may accomplish more and be more cost-effective in older people.

Comprehensive clinical benefits

Stroke and complications related to peripheral artery disease are also significantly improved with lipid-lowering, as are most cardiological procedural interventions. Importantly atheromatous plaques may become stabilised more readily through depletion of their lipid.

Comprehensive screening

All adults possibly to the age of 75, if healthy, should be screened for dyslipidaemia at intervals that depend on the total risk profile.

Which lipids?

Adequate information to manage most patients is obtained through current practice: fasting-state plasma total cholesterol and triglyceride and HDL cholesterol; calculation of LDL cholesterol is essential and generally included in the report. *Ratios of HDL to LDL or to total cholesterol have limited practical value and can confuse.*

Understanding the principles of managing dyslipidaemias
Profile of dyslipidaemias

The five major dyslipidaemias of consequence are:

1 polygenic hypercholesterolaemia, where suboptimal regulation of cholesterol or LDL metabolism predisposes the individual to a lifestyle-induced rise in plasma lipids. Inappropriate eating habits and being overweight are common and often major causes. Initial management should therefore always include an

adequate (3-month) period of properly explained dietary and other lifestyle changes. Drug intervention can usually be postponed for longer periods with safety.

2 mixed or combined hyperlipidaemia, which is analogous to the scenario above, but also involves abnormal regulation of triglyceride or VLDL metabolism. Being overweight and dietary causes including alcohol excess are very common and should be managed first.

3 familial hypercholesterolaemia, which generally has higher levels than for 1 or 2; the risk for clinical CHD is also greater, demanding more vigorous intervention especially in women after the menopause and in men after the age of about 35 years, the risk being relatively low premenopausally and in young people. Whereas dietary changes can produce some LDL cholesterol reduction, cholesterol levels above 8 mmol/L should be lowered pharmacologically as soon as the high value is confirmed, especially in the presence of other risk factors.

4 familial combined hyperlipoproteinaemia, which is commoner than 3 and one of the common dyslipidaemias in younger people with CHD. Both cholesterol (LDL) and triglyceride (VLDL and remnants of chylomicrons) are raised and HDL cholesterol is mostly low. The lipid profile can fluctuate: sometimes LDL predominates and sometimes VLDL (triglyceride), generally reflecting changes in environmental factors (weight gain and so on).

5 high triglyceride-low HDL cholesterol phenotype, which is seen increasingly as part of the overweight-insulin resistance syndrome. Although the LDL concentration is mostly normal and can even be low, the type of LDL particle, small and dense, may be more atherogenic.

Do lipoproteins matter?

The four common dyslipidaemias have one thing in common: the abnormalities are in the regulation of the lipoproteins that characterise them.

Further, the body deals with the complex interactions of all lipoproteins and our tests that focus on individual lipids underestimate the many interrelated processes that give rise to abnormal values. Does that matter? *Unexpected responses and failure to lower lipids adequately often reflect the changing balance in lipoprotein regulation that follows therapy.* For instance, LDL (or total cholesterol) may rise when combined hyperlipoproteinaemia is treated with a fibrate; or HDL cholesterol will not rise as expected. The nature and severity of the disordered regulation (mostly due to genetic factors) will determine the response to treatment; two identical lipid profiles may respond quite differently. So don't necessarily suspect the patient!

Identification of secondary causes of dyslipidaemia

Diabetes mellitus and even insulin resistance associated with being overweight are probably the commonest primary disorders causing secondary dyslipidaemia, mostly the high-triglyceride low-HDL phenotype. Renal disease poses few problems, but hypothyroidism, especially in older women, is often overlooked. Mild hypertriglyceridaemia in women on HRT is probably of little consequence.

Do less common lipoproteins need investigating?

Lp(a) has been recognised as a potential atherogenic lipoprotein if raised, especially when associated with high LDL cholesterol. It is mainly genetically determined and worth testing when other risk factors are clearly normal. It responds to very few drugs but notably to oestrogens after menopause. The protein E that is present in triglyceride-rich lipoproteins has several genotypes, one of which is apoE2, giving rise to a form of combined hyperlipoproteinaemia known as Type 3 which is highly atherogenic but usually responsive to statins and fibrates.

The role of genes

Virtually all dyslipidaemias have a genetic, generally polygenic influence. The probable balance of environmental to genetic factors should be attempted from family history, clinical stigmata of familial hypercholesterolaemia or FH (eccentric corneal arcus, thickened Achilles tendons), and often from the severity of the dyslipidaemia. FH is the only common monogenic dyslipidaemia. However, the genetic contribution to moderate 'grass-roots' high LDL is at least 25% and some believe greater; for HDL cholesterol it is at least 50%. *The extent of the genetic contribution will influence the ease with which treatment succeeds.* That works both ways. If being overweight and having dietary saturated fat are important determinants but are not modified, drugs become less effective. By contrast, complex genetic disorders such as familial combined hyperlipoproteinaemia can be resistant to therapy.

Isolated low HDL cholesterol is mostly genetic; in the absence of a satisfactory drug that raises HDL substantially, the principle is to lower LDL cholesterol to target levels.

Whom to test?

This is no longer as contentious since all adults should be tested. However, *in certain categories of patient it is virtually mandatory*:

- Patients with existing CHD and/or with other vascular atheromatous disorders
- People with multiple risk factors
- Subjects with strong family history of raised lipids or premature CHD
- Diabetics in whom dyslipidaemia is very common
- Patients with renal disease in whom dyslipidaemia contributes to adverse cardiovascular outcomes.

Other categories are better managed if their lipid profile is known—for instance, menopausal women, people with abdominal obesity, and people who drink alcohol excessively.

Why is absolute risk important?

These calculations are based on prospective trials such as Framingham and therefore include risk factors that had been studied. Unmodifiable factors include family history, age and gender; modifiable factors include plasma lipids, blood pressure, and the patient's smoking status. From these are calculated the probable risk of a clinical event from CHD over the following 10 years. That usually focuses a patient's attention. The probability is high for an older person with several risk factors. For a young person aged 20, even the presence of FH in the absence of other factors carries a low risk that may not justify pharmacological intervention. *Advice in the U.K. is to initiate drug therapy when the 10-year risk exceeds 15%; the European guideline is 20%.* These appear to be reasonable numbers.

Implementing principles of treatment

This is not a guide to detailed therapy but several of the above principles are worth emphasising:

- Establish the nature of the lipid disorder.
- Assess the total risk.
- Determine the target for LDL cholesterol, triglyceride and HDL cholesterol from Pharmaceutical Benefits Scheme (PBS) guidelines for lipid lowering or the slightly more aggressive *NHF lipid management guidelines.*
- Maximise non-pharmacological interventions first and throughout. Weight loss of a few kilograms improves the responsiveness to drugs.
- If absolute risk remains high, initiate drug therapy at levels of lipids shown in the guidelines.
- Aim to have patients reach target levels.
- Strive to have the patient maintain compliance.
- Consider ancillary treatments such as aspirin in severely dyslipidaemic older patients, an antioxidant like vitamin E, and fish oil, recently shown to be effective in a secondary prevention trial. Folate, which is cheap and safe, may soon be added.
- Test relatives of all dyslipidaemic patients.

Comments on pharmacotherapy

- The advent of statins has greatly eased management primarily of hypercholesterolaemia and of combined hyperlipidaemia when excess LDL predominates.
- The limitation of fibrate choice (gemfibrozil being less effective than some) makes management of combined hyperlipidaemias in which triglycerides predominate often difficult.
- Combining statins and fibrates has not been as problematical as originally envisaged and is mostly effective in combined dyslipidaemia.
- Fish oils added to a fibrate for lowering triglyceride levels can be effective.
- Adding small amounts of a bile acid-sequestering resin to a statin is useful for reaching LDL cholesterol targets.
- Nicotinic acid is still an excellent drug, especially for intractable combined hyperlipidaemia and for severe

hypertriglyceridaemia. Some patients tolerate the side effect of flushing by taking aspirin simultaneously.

■ Newer drugs that inhibit cholesterol absorption and more acceptable bile acid-sequestering drugs are in late trial stage.

BIBLIOGRAPHY

Gotto A. M., Whitney E., Stein E. A. et al. Relation between baseline and on-treatment lipid parameters and first acute major coronary events in the Air Force / Texas Coronary Atherosclerosis Prevention Study (AFCAPS/TexCAPS). *Circulation* 2000; 201: 477–84.

LIPID Study Group. Long-term intervention with pravastatin in ischemic coronary disease (LIPID) study. *N Engl J Med* 1998; 339: 1349–57.

Pedersen T. R., Olsson A. G., Faergeman O. et al. Lipoprotein changes and reduction in the incidence of major coronary heart disease events in the 4S study. *Circulation* 1998; 97: 1453–60.

Rubins H. B., Robins S. J., Collins D. et al. Gemfibrozil for the secondary prevention of coronary heart disease in men with low levels of high density lipoprotein cholesterol. *N Engl J Med* 1999; 341: 410–8.

Sacks F. M., Moye L. A., Davis B. R. et al. Relationship between plasma LDL concentrations during treatment with pravastatin and recurrent coronary events in the cholesterol and recurrent events trial. *Circulation* 1998; 97: 1446–52.

West of Scotland Primary Prevention Study Group. Influence of pravastatin and plasma lipids on clinical events in the WOSCOPS study. *Circulation* 1998; 97: 1440–5.

Interpretation and significance of a high blood cholesterol

8

A. M. Dart, C. Reid, G. L. Jennings, R. A. J. Conyers and E. M. Nicholls

SYNOPSIS

The interpretation of blood cholesterol measurements requires an understanding of the magnitude and causes of their biological and analytical variability. Recommendations for limiting such variability include blood sampling under standard conditions and the use of laboratories performing acceptably in National Quality Assurance Programs. Even with these precautions, management decisions should only be made on the mean results of at least two samples, differing by no more than 0.75 mmol/L.

Introduction

It is important for physicians to be aware of possible pitfalls in the interpretation of cholesterol (and triglyceride) measurements and to appreciate the causes of variability and the ways in which these may be minimised. This article will cover measurement of total cholesterol, HDL cholesterol and triglycerides. *Interpretation of a high cholesterol concentration in the presence of a high triglycerides concentration (> 5.0 mmol/L) can be difficult.* In such circumstances, it is usually best to reconsider the significance of cholesterol values after triglyceride values have been lowered.

Since in routine rather than research laboratories measurements are made of total cholesterol, HDL cholesterol and triglyceride, reference will be made to these, although it must be realised that the pathologically relevant fraction is LDL cholesterol. This is generally computed by the Friedewald equation as LDL cholesterol = total cholesterol – HDL – triglycerides/2.2.

Technical aspects
Total cholesterol

Analytical problems in total cholesterol measurement stem from two aspects of all laboratory measurements:

1 Precision—this relates to the variability of repeated measurements of the same sample using the same method. Precision, or, more correctly, imprecision, is reported as the coefficient of variation (CV). This is calculated as standard deviation/mean x 100, and is a measure of the dispersion of results about their mean. For cholesterol measurements, a CV of ±5% is currently achievable and a goal of ±3% or better is desirable.

2 Bias—this relates to the divergence between the value assigned to a sample by the method in use and the 'true value' or 'gold standard' value determined by some other generally accepted reference method. Bias in routine clinical measurement of total cholesterol should not exceed 5%.

The effects of different levels of precision and bias are shown in Figure 8.1 and relate to the measurement of a single serum sample with a true total cholesterol concentration of 6 mmol/L. If such a sample is analysed 100 times in a laboratory with a bias of +5% and a CV of ±5%, then in 95 of these estimations that result will be between 5.7 and 6.9 mmol/L. In the remaining five analyses, the result would be likely to be outside these limits. In a laboratory with a bias of –5% (not shown), the corresponding 95% confidence limits would be 5.1 and 6.3 mmol/L. In all these instances, any contribution from biological variability is ignored.

Routine cholesterol measurement utilises the enzymatic conversion of cholesterol with the formation of hydrogen peroxide, which can be determined by an associated photometric change. Calibrators are required to convert the measurement of physical change (e.g. optical density change) to cholesterol concentration. Once calibrated, the performance of an assay can

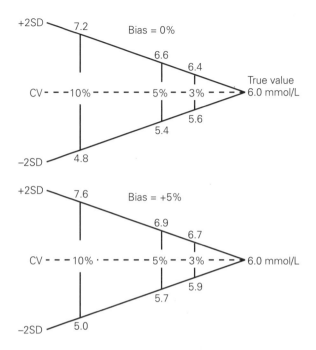

FIGURE 8.1 The effects of different levels of precision (CV) and bias on the measurement of total cholesterol of serum with a true cholesterol concentration of 6 mmol/L

be monitored by using a quality control (QC) sample. The Royal College of Pathologists of Australasia and the Australian Association of Clinical Biochemists have established the Australian Quality Assurance Program (RCPA-AACB-AQAP). The QC sample produced for this program is analysed by a direct chemical method. Participating laboratories receive frozen aliquots and report their findings back to AQAP. In turn, the participating laboratories are informed of their performance as well as that of other participating laboratories.

HDL cholesterol

HDL cholesterol is usually measured by precipitation of apolipoprotein B containing lipoproteins (LDL, VLDL) followed by determination of the cholesterol concentration in the non-precipitated fraction. Measurement errors can thus arise both from the final cholesterol measurement as well as from inadequate precipitation. The latter is a particular problem with hypertriglyceridaemic samples (particularly above 5 mmol/L). The supernatant should be inspected to ensure that it is clear.

Triglycerides

Most methods for triglyceride measurement rely on the conversion of triglyceride to free glycerol, which is subsequently determined. Free glycerol is, however, present in blood and available methods vary as to whether or not 'glycerol blanking' occurs (i.e. the estimation of free glycerol before triglyceride hydrolysis).

Physiological aspects
Cholesterol

Even if samples were always measured with complete (100%) accuracy (*supra vide*), variation would be found on measuring repeat samples from the same subject. Several factors contribute to this variability, which is present despite overnight fasting or abstinence from food for several hours.

Posture

Blood samples withdrawn in the standing position have higher cholesterol concentrations than those taken with the patients recumbent. Samples should be taken after several minutes' seated or supine rest.

Venous/capillary blood samples

Prolonged venous stasis leads to elevated cholesterol concentrations and should be avoided. Capillary and venous blood cholesterol concentration can differ and therefore a consistent approach should be used.

Diurnal variation

Total cholesterol values vary both diurnally and seasonally. Lowest values are found in the early morning and highest in the evening.

Plasma/serum

Anticoagulants in collecting tubes influence cholesterol measurements to a variable degree. Serum samples are generally preferred.

Physical state

Chronic illness may depress cholesterol levels. In particular, values taken during convalescence after myocardial infarction are depressed. Measurements within 24 hours of admission or 3 months postinfarction are recommended.

Drug therapy

Both prescribed and self-administered drugs may modify cholesterol levels, although triglyceride levels are usually more affected. Interpretation of blood lipid results should be made with knowledge of a current drug history (including alcohol).

Triglycerides

Serum triglyceride values show the greatest variability of all the commonly measured lipid parameters, in large part due to a large biological variation. Accurate triglyceride levels depend on prolonged fasting and are sensitive to weight change and many medications (e.g. diuretics, alcohol, and oral contraceptives). A variety of hormones increase lipolysis and therefore free glycerol levels. In addition, levels may be raised in diabetes and liver failure. Long-term biological variability in the order of 10% has also been noted.

Is the result abnormal/positive?

The concept of abnormal or positive does not apply in any absolute sense to measurements of cholesterol and triglyceride. Rather, values of these parameters need to be considered in the light of the overall clinical picture, principally to assess the risk of macrovascular, particularly coronary, disease and to decide whether specific therapeutic agents are required.

The guidelines for treatment in a particular situation are available from several bodies, most notably the National Heart Foundation and the Pharmaceutical Benefits Scheme (PBS).

What action is needed if result is abnormal/positive?

Initial therapy for values identified as inappropriately high for the particular clinical circumstances should generally first be treated by dietary modifications and drug therapy instituted only when it is clear that dietary approaches are inadequate to achieve the required lipid levels. In addition, care needs to be taken to ensure that any such elevation is not secondary to some other underlying metabolic process. Thus, for example, an increase in cholesterol may be a manifestation of hypothyroidism; elevated triglycerides or mixed hyperlipidaemia may be found commonly in diabetes, alcohol excess and renal failure.

Once it is clear that specific pharmacological therapy is required, the appropriate choice depends on the nature of the lipid abnormality present.

Hypercholesterolaemia

This is now most commonly treated with a statin drug. Additional and/or alternative agents include questran and probucol, although this may lower HDL. Fibrates are more useful at treating mixed hyperlipidaemia.

Nicotinic acid is rather infrequently used due to an extensive side-effect profile.

Hypertriglyceridaemia and mixed hyperlipidaemia

Fish oils are particular successful in the treatment of high triglyceride levels but have little effect on cholesterol. Fibrates are an effective treatment in mixed hyperlipidaemia as is nicotinic acid. At present, there is no specific treatment available to elevate HDL cholesterol, although most cholesterol-lowering agents such as statin do produce a modest (approximately 10%) elevation. As already indicated probucol differs markedly in this respect and can be associated with a profound reduction in HDL cholesterol.

Summary

The technical and biological variation in lipid measurements, together with the fact that their reduction is rarely urgently required (possible exceptions may include severely elevated triglycerides associated with pancreatitis), mean that it is appropriate to obtain at least two and possibly more baseline measurements under standardised conditions before instituting pharmacological therapy. At the present time, there is extremely good medication available to lower total (LDL) cholesterol and effective treatment for mixed hyperlipidaemia and hypertri-glyceridaemia. Treatment for low HDL is inadequate. This will probably change in the next few years although further trials will still be required to establish that elevation of a low HDL is indeed therapeutically effective.

9 | Hyperuricaemia

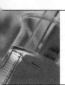

B. T. Emmerson

SYNOPSIS

When an elevated serum urate concentration is found, the cause needs to be sought. Both genetic and environmental factors will contribute. In practice, the major significant risk from hyperuricaemia is the development of gouty arthritis.

Introduction

In the apparently normal population, the distribution of serum urate concentrations is skewed towards higher values as it includes many subjects who are asymptomatic at the time but who later develop gout. Even the 95% population range includes many who will later develop gout. It is therefore difficult to define the upper limit of the 'normal' serum urate. Pragmatically, the best value to choose is the point at which there is minimal overlap between the curves of the distribution of the serum urate concentration range in the healthy population compared with that in a population with gout. This overlap occurs at a value of approximately 0.42 mmol/L in males and 0.36 mmol/L in females. Approximately 7% of the apparently normal male population has serum urate concentrations greater than these values. These values are internationally accepted and provide useful bases for interpreting the clinical significance of hyperuricaemia.

The serum urate rises in normal males at puberty by approximately 0.06 mmol/L and in normal females at the menopause by a similar amount. The annual risk of acute gout in a patient with a serum urate concentration of 0.54 mmol/L is approximately 5% or 1 in 20. This risk does not justify the treatment of asymptomatic hyperuricaemia, although it would do so in someone who had already suffered acute attacks of gout. This reassurance does not necessarily carry over to patients with persistent hyperuricaemia greater than 0.6 mmol/L.

Technical aspects

Current autoanalyser techniques for measuring the serum urate concentration in both serum and urine can be regarded as being reliable for all clinical purposes.

Physiological aspects

Hyperuricaemia results from an imbalance between production and excretion of urate. Urate is principally produced by *de novo* nucleoprotein production and metabolism, from dietary purine consumption and by the degradation of ATP within the body at a rate faster than can be reutilised. Two-thirds of the urate which is produced is excreted in the urine and one-third is eliminated in intestinal secretions by a passive process.

The elimination of urate by the kidney is determined by the renal clearance of urate which is principally under genetic control (Table 9.1). There is, however, a wide range in the normal urate clearance (between 4 and 14 mL/minute) and this leads to a wide variation in the ability of apparently normal subjects to eliminate urate by the renal route. A number of different racial groups in the Pacific area appear to have inherited a reduced ability to excrete urate, as reflected by a reduced urate clearance. Renal excretion of urate is also modified by a variety of conditions, including the presence of renal disease, the consumption of drugs which retain urate (such as thiazide diuretics or low dose salicylate therapy), by the effect of lactate, ketones or angiotensin on the kidney tubule, by hypertension, and by any factors which cause plasma volume concentration or a urine volume of less than 1 mL per minute. Hyperuricaemia can also result from an increase in the production of urate, particularly when it is not matched by an increase in renal excretion. Thus a high purine diet (particularly one containing much flesh or nuclear material) will contribute, as will the consumption of alcoholic beverages. This occurs firstly because the alcohol is metabolised to lactate which acts to reduce the renal excretion of urate; secondly because it increases ATP degradation to AMP and the purine bases; and thirdly because of the purines which originate in yeast and which are contained in beer. Obesity is also associated with both increased production and reduced excretion of urate and is a common contributor to hyperuricaemia. The common pattern in this country of regular beer consumption associated with obesity, hypertriglyceridaemia and the insulin resistance syndrome is also frequently associated with the development of hyperuricaemia and gout.

TABLE 9.1 Common causes of sustained hyperuricaemia

1 Inherited reduction in urate excretion
Low urate clearance in an otherwise normal kidney

2 Acquired reduction in urate excretion
Drugs	-	thiazide diuretics
	-	low dose salicylate
Metabolites	-	lactate
	-	ketones
	-	angiotensin
	-	vasopressin
Renal	-	plasma-volume contraction
	-	hypertension
	-	reduced urine volume (<1 mL/min)

3 Acquired increase in urate production
High purine (nucleoprotein) intake
Regular alcohol consumption
Obesity and hypertriglyceridaemia
Tissue hypoxia due to systemic disease
Myelopoliferative disorders

Many of the factors contributing to hyperuricaemia can be corrected when identified, and this can lead to a fall in the serum urate concentration to within the normal range. However, this approach does require considerable motivation on the part of the patient. Any weight loss should be gradual. Weight loss should never be sufficient to induce ketosis which would reduce the renal excretion of urate and aggravate the hyperuricaemia.

Is the result abnormal?

If the cause of the hyperuricaemia is not apparent from the clinical assessment of the history and examination of the patient, it can be investigated by measuring the fall in the serum and urine urate concentration after 1 week of dietary purine restriction. This will give an indication of the contribution of the patient's diet to the hyperuricaemia and allow the urate clearance to be calculated, as well as the 24-hour urinary urate excretion on a low purine diet. If this value is greater than 4 mmol/24 hours on a low purine diet, then excessive production of urate is suggested, indicating the need to use xanthine oxidase inhibiting drugs.

What action is needed if the result is abnormal?

The cause of hyperuricaemia can be determined either from the history and examination alone or by the investigations already suggested. Many of these causes can be corrected. If the recurrent gout is present, however, and the patient feels that prevention of further attacks is justified by regular medication, then therapy with urate-lowering drugs is desirable. The goal should be to have a serum urate persistently below 0.36 mmol/L, and the dose of drug given (either a xanthine oxidase inhibitor or a uricosuric agent) should be adjusted to achieve this goal.

Summary

The principal complications of hyperuricaemia are gout and renal colic. Simple clinical and laboratory assessment can usually identify factors contributing to the hyperuricaemia and attention can then be paid to their correction. If this is insufficient, and gout remains a problem, urate-lowering drugs can be given on a regular basis and this should prevent future adverse effects. Asymptomatic hyperuricaemia should be regarded as an associated disorder, the cause of which should be sought and corrected where possible. It should rarely be treated with medication.

FURTHER READING

Emmerson B. T. *Getting Rid of Gout—A Guide to Management & Prevention*. Melbourne: Oxford University Press, 1996.

Emmerson B. T. Hyperuricaemia and gout. In: Noe D. A. and Rock R. C., eds. *Laboratory Medicine—the Detection and Interpretation of Clinical Laboratory Studies*. Philadelphia: Williams & Wilkins, 1994.

Emmerson B. T. Identification of the causes of persistent hyperuricaemia. *Lancet* 1991; 337: 1461–3.

Emmerson B. T. The management of gout. *N Engl J Med* 1996; 334: 445–51.

Liver function tests

L. W. Powell, M. L. Bassett and W. G. E. Cooksley

Introduction

An almost bewildering array of liver function tests is available for assessing the patient with suspected liver disease. Many of these are currently included in routine biochemical screens, and clinicians are faced with an increasing number of abnormal tests to interpret. Fortunately in the last decade the tests in the biochemical screens have become standardised, enabling an easier interpretation of results. This review is designed to help the clinician assess, in particular, abnormal first-line screening tests and to determine when more expensive and specialised second-line biochemical or radiological and scanning procedures are required.

Liver function tests

Liver function tests often included in SMAC profiles include total bilirubin, conjugated bilirubin, alkaline phosphatase, alanine transaminase, aspartate transaminase, gamma glutamyl transpeptidase, serum albumin and serum globulin.

The term 'liver function tests' is really a misnomer, as few of these investigations really assess liver function; most are based on some property of the damaged hepatocyte or bile canaliculus. Nowadays, with increasing use of liver transplantation, there is a need to assess liver function. Thus, hepatologists usually distinguish between tests of hepatocyte damage (transaminases or, in the case of biliary tract disorders, tests of cholestasis) and tests of synthetic function which include albumin and the measurement of prothrombin time. Many of the tests lack specificity. For example, elevated serum bilirubin or enzyme levels are encountered not infrequently in patients without primary liver disease (e.g. those with infection, trauma and cardiac failure). The difficulty arises in determining the probability of the presence of underlying liver disease and the need to pursue the abnormal result further.

A rational and accurate interpretation of liver function tests requires a minimum knowledge of the relevant physiology and biochemistry. A discussion of this is outside the scope of the present article and interested readers are referred to standard texts.[1, 2] However, several points warrant particular emphasis.

Is the result abnormal?
Serum bilirubin

In patients with normal enzymes and unexplained elevation of serum total bilirubin, both conjugated and unconjugated fractions should be measured. This is important in the early detection of disorders associated with predominantly unconjugated hyperbilirubinaemia (e.g. Gilbert's syndrome, haemolysis) and in differentiating them from hepatobiliary diseases. This distinction may avoid much unnecessary investigation and anxiety on the part of both patient and doctor. Bilirubin in the urine occurs only when the serum-conjugated bilirubin is raised and always indicates hepatobiliary disease.

Serum transaminases

Serum aspartate aminotransaminase (AST or SGOT)
This aminotransferase enzyme is present in high concentration in the hepatocyte but it is also present in the heart, skeletal muscle and kidney. Leakage into the circulation occurs following changes in cell permeability due to ischaemia or necrosis. Thus elevated serum levels are encountered frequently in ischaemic heart disease and with muscle injury (e.g. after intramuscular injections).

The highest AST levels are found in acute viral hepatitis and drug hepatitis (e.g. paracetamol overdose), when levels are frequently in excess of 1000 U/L. However, there is only a crude quantitative correlation between serum levels and the extent of liver necrosis, and the height of the elevation is not a useful index of either severity or prognosis. A persistently elevated AST level 3 months after an attack of viral hepatitis suggests chronic hepatitis, and is an indication for further investigation, including liver biopsy. Lesser degrees of transaminase elevation are seen in many hepatobiliary diseases, such as alcoholic and drug hepatitis, chronic active hepatitis, intrahepatic and extrahepatic cholestasis, and hepatic neoplasms.

Serum alamine aminotransferase (ALT or SGPT)

This enzyme is more specific for liver and is now routinely included in multiple biochemical analyses. The level is usually higher than the AST with one important exception—acute alcoholic hepatitis where the ALT/AST ratio may be 1 or less. In milder forms of liver injury, the ALT level may be abnormal when the AST is still within the normal range. As patients progress from chronic hepatitis to cirrhosis, the ALT /AST ratio will gradually reverse and in patients with cirrhosis the AST is often higher.

Serum alkaline phosphatase (AP)

This enzyme arises primarily from liver, bone and placenta. Hepatic alkaline phosphatase is associated with the biliary canalicular microvilli. Marked elevations are characteristic of intrahepatic cholestasis and extrahepatic obstruction although lesser elevations occur in many types of liver diseases. Alkaline phosphatase of bony origin may be distinguished from hepatic alkaline phosphatase by measuring serum 5'nucleotidase (5NT) which is specific for liver disease but, if the gamma-glutamyl transpeptidase is also elevated, it is likely that the alkaline phosphatase originates from the hepatobiliary system.

Serum gamma-glutamyl transpeptidase (GGT)

GGT is found mainly in liver, kidney and muscle. It is a microsomal enzyme and increased serum levels occur following microsomal induction, particularly by alcohol, herbal remedies and drugs as well as microsomal injury from any cause. The main clinical applications of GGT levels are as a sensitive index of early liver disease or of continued heavy drinking in alcoholism.

Serum albumin

Albumin is synthesised exclusively by the liver. A low serum albumin may reflect chronic impairment of albumin synthesis by the liver, although other causes such as shifts in albumin or fluid between compartments also alter serum albumin. A low serum albumin due to liver disease usually indicates a chronic disease process. In contrast, the prothrombin time will be prolonged at an earlier stage of liver failure because of the shorter half-life of the coagulation factors synthesised by the liver. The liver is the major site of synthesis of many coagulation factors. In addition, vitamin K malabsorption (e.g. complicating severe or prolonged cholestasis) will reduce the synthesis of vitamin K-dependent factors II, VII, IX and X. Thus, serum albumin and prothrombin time can be regarded as useful tests of liver function. Serum immunoglobulins are not tests of liver function. The levels are often non-specifically elevated in liver disease, particularly in chronic autoimmune liver diseases.

What action is needed if the result is abnormal?

There are two situations that may be encountered clinically.

The serum bilirubin level is elevated but the enzyme levels are normal

In this situation one should recheck the history with a few specific questions. Does the patient suffer from non-hepatic illness (e.g. cardiac failure) which may affect hepatic handling or bilirubin? Is there a family history of haemolytic disease (e.g. thalassaemia) or of congenital disorders (e.g. Gilbert's syndrome)? Is the elevated serum bilirubin level predominantly conjugated or unconjugated?

It is worth noting that significant liver disease is rarely present if elevation of the serum bilirubin is the only persistent abnormality.

The serum enzymes are elevated with or without elevation of the serum bilirubin level

In this situation an appropriate procedure is as follows:
1 Check the history for symptoms suggesting acute or chronic viral hepatitis, and for exposure to medication (prescription, over-the-counter, and alternative therapy), and especially

excessive alcohol intake. Some patients develop hepatic damage when taking as little as 40 g of ethanol (approximately four drinks per day), although most patients with alcoholic liver disease consume at least 100 g ethanol daily (approximately 10 standard drinks per day). Although it is common knowledge that heavy drinkers frequently underestimate their alcohol intake, it is surprising how often alcoholic liver disease is overlooked as a diagnosis. Similarly, as more and more medications are introduced, it becomes increasingly difficult to predict hepatotoxicity and the medical practitioner needs to have available a comprehensive list of the side effects of all medications. Hepatotoxicity due to medications usually appears within the first 3 months of commencement of the medication, but there are some notable exceptions (e.g. methotrexate). If in doubt, the suspected drug should be stopped, particularly if alternative therapy is available.

2 Repeat the test on a further occasion, to confirm the presence of a persistent abnormality before proceeding further.

3 Look for other non-hepatic conditions that may cause abnormal liver function tests, such as obesity (may be associated with non-alcoholic steatohepatitis), cardiac failure, chronic infections, thyrotoxicosis, diabetes mellitus, inflammatory bowel disease, coeliac disease, connective tissue diseases, haematological malignancies and disseminated malignancy. Arrange appropriate investigations depending on the degree of clinical suspicion.

4 If persistent and unexplained elevation is present, further (second- or third-line) investigations are indicated to determine the aetiology of the disorder. At this stage the clinician should make a conscious distinction between hepatocellular or cholestatic liver disease although in many cases, particularly with medication-induced liver injury, a mixed hepatocellular-cholestatic picture is present.

Hepatocellular or mixed hepatocellular-cholestatic pattern

If the abnormalities point to hepatocellular or mixed hepatocellular-cholestatic disease, the most helpful definitive investigation is liver biopsy. An ultrasound of the liver should usually be performed first to look for evidence of malignancy (primary or secondary), increased echogenicity (suggestive but not diagnostic of fatty infiltration) and evidence of cirrhosis and portal hypertension. Complementary tests which are helpful in determining aetiology, and in some cases may give a firm diagnosis without the need for liver biopsy, include:

- serology for hepatitis A, B, C, Epstein-Barr virus and cytomegalovirus
- tissue autoantibodies (antinuclear, smooth muscle and mitochondrial antibodies)
- transferrin saturation (ratio of serum iron and TIBC) and serum ferritin levels and, if these are abnormal, HFE mutations (C282Y and H63D) for haemochromatosis
- fasting triglyceride and glucose levels
- serum copper and ceruloplasmin levels
- serum alpha 1-antitrypsin levels
- serum alpha-fetoprotein (for primary hepatocellular carcinoma).

With increasing prevalence of chronic viral hepatitis and the availability of multiple different assays, confusion may occur as a result of a request for 'hepatitis serology' not covering the desired investigations. This is because the Medicare item numbers cover different clusters of tests:

- Tests for acute hepatitis—IgM antibodies against hepatitis A virus and hepatitis B virus (antiHBc). There is no assay for IgM against hepatitis C virus and, since IgG assay for hepatitis C may take a month or two to become positive, measurement of virus (PCR for HCV RNA) is necessary. HBsAg is also usually done.
- Tests for chronic hepatitis—HbsAg and IgG antibodies against hepatitis B virus (antiHBc) and hepatitis C. Antibodies against HDV and HEV will be carried out in appropriate circumstances.
- Preimmunisation status—IgG antibodies against HAV and HBV.

Cholestatic pattern

If the abnormalities point to a cholestatic disease process (predominant elevation of the serum AP with or without elevated conjugated bilirubin) one must distinguish between mechanical obstruction of the bile ducts and intrahepatic cholestasis. Ultrasound examination of the liver and biliary tree is the initial investigation of choice. Computerised tomography is useful in the assessment of possible tumours (e.g. pancreas, primary and secondary hepatic). If dilated bile ducts are demonstrated, one should proceed to more definitive radiological investigations such as cholangiography (either magnetic resonance imaging (MRI), retrograde or percutaneous cholangiopancreatography) to demonstrate the cause and site of the obstruction. If ultrasound examination does not confirm the presence of dilated bile ducts, percutaneous needle biopsy of the liver is usually recommended. In primary sclerosing cholangitis the bile ducts may not be dilated on ultrasound but MRI may avoid the need for cholangiography.

Summary

Few areas of clinical medicine illustrate better the need for a thorough history and careful clinical examination than the investigation of suspected hepatobiliary disease. Although sophisticated tests such as endoscopic retrograde cholangiopancreatography (ERCP), magnetic resonance cholangiopancreatography (MRCP) and liver biopsy often enable a precise diagnosis, their inappropriate use without proper integration with the clinical findings may result in unnecessary expense and misdiagnoses. It is also important to advise patients that investigation of hepatobiliary disease may involve a small amount of risk, particularly if either liver biopsy or ERCP is required. These investigations should be performed by experienced medical practitioners after other measures have failed to give a firm diagnosis, and with full discussion of the benefits and possible complications. Despite the potential for complications, they are extremely useful investigations when used appropriately.

REFERENCES

1 Isselbacher K. J., Braunwald E., Wilson J. D., Martin I. II, Fauci A. S. and Kasper D. L., eds. *Harrison's Principles of Internal Medicine.* 15th edn. New York: McGraw-Hill, 2001.

2 Kaplan M. M. Laboratory tests. In: Schiff L. and Schiff E. R. *Diseases of the Liver.*
7th edn. New York: Lippincott, 1993, pp. 108–44.

11 | The glucose tolerance test

S. K. Gan and D. J. Chisholm

SYNOPSIS

The role of the oral glucose tolerance test (OGTT) has evolved over recent years with the use of a lower fasting glucose threshold for the diagnosis of diabetes and the introduction of a new category, 'impaired fasting glucose', in the classification of glucose tolerance. Use of the new lower diagnostic threshold for the fasting venous plasma glucose alone (≥ 7.0 mmol/L) is reasonably specific for diabetes but subjects with lower fasting levels may be misclassified without an OGTT. Therefore the 2-hour post glucose load reading in a glucose tolerance test continues to have a role in the diagnosis of diabetes, although limited to certain clinical situations. The future place of the test in the diagnosis of diabetes will continue to be modified as further data become available.

Introduction

The use of the OGTT in the diagnosis and classification of glucose intolerance and diabetes mellitus has recently undergone revision. In particular, a lower fasting glucose threshold has been used for the diagnosis of diabetes mellitus by both the American Diabetes Association (ADA) and the World Health Organisation

(WHO) to enhance the diagnostic sensitivity of the fasting glucose level. This is supported by recent data on the risk of diabetic complications in relation to glucose levels. There has been doubt, however, that the fasting glucose should replace the OGTT (as recommended by the ADA) and a continued role for the test has been reflected in the recent position statements of the WHO and the Australasian Working Party on Diagnostic Criteria for Diabetes Mellitus. The final report by the WHO is, however, still awaited.

The categories of glucose tolerance are currently defined as:

1 normal
2 impaired fasting glucose (IFG)
3 impaired glucose tolerance (IGT)
4 diabetes mellitus.

The diagnosis of IGT does not indicate a necessary progression to diabetes—in fact, only about 20% of subjects with IGT develop diabetes mellitus and many revert to a normal glucose tolerance test. Significantly, the category of IGT is associated with other manifestations of the metabolic syndrome and an increased risk of cardiovascular disease. There are currently insufficient data to be certain if the new category of IFG is associated with the same risk status as IGT (although there are some similarities in risk) and further data are awaited.

Technical aspects

Subjects should receive a relatively high carbohydrate diet (at least 150 g) for 3 days before the test. On the morning of the test, 75 g glucose (or 1.75 g/kg up to 75 g in children) is given, following an overnight fast. Blood samples are taken while fasting and 2 hours after the glucose load.

Care must be taken to distinguish between glucose levels performed on plasma or blood (plasma levels are approximately 13% higher than whole blood levels) and capillary or venous samples (capillary is higher in the non-fasting state). Venous samples are normally taken during an OGTT. It should be noted that glucose preservatives (e.g. fluoride oxalate) reduce but do not totally prevent glycolysis during sample transport/holding; this can lead to underestimation of the true glucose concentrations.

Physiological aspects

The OGTT is a relatively imprecise test as biological variation in the response to glucose ingestion is added to any assay error. Where a single glucose level, other than the fasting level, slightly exceeds the normal, the result of the test should probably be regarded as normal.

If the test has been performed during severe stress or intercurrent illness, mild elevations of blood glucose levels should not be diagnosed as diabetes until the test is repeated under more normal circumstances.

Undue carbohydrate restriction on the days prior to the test can lead to an impairment of glucose tolerance.

A 'flat' glucose tolerance curve (low peak level) has sometimes been regarded as indicative of malabsorption. However, a flat curve is a fairly common finding in fit, normal people with very efficient glucose disposal.

It has become evident that some individuals can have an impaired fasting plasma glucose but the 2-hour post glucose load level may be in the diabetic range. A diabetic glucose tolerance test response, however, is rare if the fasting venous plasma glucose is less than 5.5 mmol/L. An abnormal fasting plasma glucose with a normal 2-hour level may also occur and some of these variabilities appear to reflect different population backgrounds.

Is the result abnormal?

The current diagnostic criteria as set out by the ADS Position Statement are shown in Table 11.1.

It should be stressed that the OGTT is usually *not* necessary in the diagnosis of diabetes mellitus. Either a fasting venous plasma glucose above 7.0 mmol/L (blood glucose > 6.1 mmol/L) or a random plasma glucose above 11.1 mmol/L (blood glucose > 10 mmol/L) if repeated, establishes a definite diagnosis of diabetes mellitus. Nearly all subjects who have symptomatic hyperglycaemia will easily exceed these cut-off points, and even asymptomatic patients with glycosuria will generally have glucose levels in the diagnostic range if they do have diabetes.

If a diagnosis of diabetes is suspected and fasting venous plasma glucose is between 5.5 and 7.0 mmol/L (a diabetic OGTT

TABLE 11.1 Values for diagnosis of diabetes mellitus and other categories of hyperglycaemia

	GLUCOSE CONCENTRATION (mmol/L)	
	PLASMA *(whole blood)*	
	Venous	**Capillary**
DIABETES MELLITUS Fasting	≥ 7.0 (≥6.1)	≥ 7.0 (≥6.1)
‖ 2 h post glucose load or both	≥ 11.1 (≥10.0)	≥ 12.2 (≥11.1)
IMPAIRED GLUCOSE TOLERANCE (IGT) Fasting (if measured)	< 7.0 (<6.1)	< 7.0 (<6.1)
and 2 h post glucose load	≥ 7.8 (≥6.7) and < 11.1 (<10.0)	≥ 8.9 (≥7.8) and < 12.2 (<11.1)
IMPAIRED FASTING GLYCAEMIA (IFG) Fasting	≥ 6.1 (≥5.6) and < 7.0 (<6.1)	≥ 6.1 (≥5.6) and < 7.0 (<6.1)
2 h post glucose load (if measured)	< 7.8 (<6.7)	< 8.9 (<7.8)
NORMAL Fasting	< 6.1 (<5.6)	< 6.1 (<5.6)
2 h post glucose load (if measured)	< 7.8 (<6.7)	< 8.9 (<7.8)

is very unlikely with a fasting plasma glucose less than 5.5 mmol) or random plasma glucose is less than 11.1 mmol/L, an OGTT is appropriate.

Unfortunately, an OGTT is often requested inappropriately, especially in the following three situations:

1 A newly presenting patient with symptoms of hyperglycaemia or substantial glycosuria (this includes nearly all children). The correct procedure here is to determine a fasting or random plasma glucose level which will nearly always establish the diagnosis. The performance of an OGTT is unnecessary and will delay appropriate therapy.

2 A patient with diabetes—an OGTT should not be used to determine the type of therapy or the response to therapy in diabetes.

3 A patient under stress, with intercurrent illness or taking medications that induce elevated blood glucose levels—an OGTT should not be performed at times of severe physical or emotional stress or intercurrent illness, or in patients on medications (e.g. corticosteroids) which may elevate blood glucose levels. If diabetes mellitus is present in these situations a fasting or random blood glucose level will be elevated.

What to do about a diagnosis of impaired glucose tolerance

There is no uniformity of opinion about the clinical approach to this situation but we recommend the following guidelines:

■ If there is a definite family history of non-insulin-dependent diabetes, advise the patient to follow an appropriate diabetic diet and maintain a good level of physical activity but do *not* label the patient with the diagnosis of 'diabetes' or 'early diabetes' (which may prejudice insurance, superannuation, etc.). Warn them of the symptoms of hyperglycaemia and check a fasting glucose level at 6–12 month intervals.

■ If there is not a definite family history of diabetes, warn the person that there is an approximate 20% risk of developing diabetes. Offer the suggestion of reducing this chance by restriction of free sugar and fat intake plus regular exercise; aim for weight reduction if they are obese. Warn them of the symptoms of hyperglycaemia and check a fasting glucose level at 6–12 monthly intervals.

■ If the person is pregnant, a diabetic diet should be followed and blood glucose levels monitored. It should be noted that epidemiological data suggest that even slight hyperglycaemia represents a risk to the foetus during pregnancy. Thus, the patient should be treated as having diabetes for the duration of the pregnancy.

The above advice should be tempered according to the age of the subject. A diagnosis of impaired glucose tolerance at age 75 would be of much less consequence than the same diagnosis at age 40. As impaired glucose tolerance has been associated with an increase in cardiovascular risk, it is sensible to assess other cardiovascular risk factors in this situation and advise the patient accordingly.

What to do about a diagnosis of impaired fasting glucose

An OGTT should be performed to exclude the presence of diabetes and IGT if suspicion of diabetes is high. If IFG in isolation is confirmed, it may be reasonable to adopt an approach broadly similar to that with the IGT category at this point in time while further data are awaited about the precise risk status.

What to do about a diagnosis of diabetes mellitus

Decide if the diagnosis is likely to be type 1 or type 2 diabetes. Pointers to type 1 diabetes include age less than 30 years, presence of ketones in the urine, normal or reduced body weight and either (1) an absence of family history of diabetes or (2) a history of type 1 diabetes. If in doubt, measurement of antiGAD antibodies can be performed as an indicator of type 1 diabetes.

If type 1 diabetes is diagnosed, commence insulin therapy immediately.

If the diagnosis is type 2 diabetes, the prescription is diet and exercise ± sulfonylurea or biguanide tablets. Insulin is occasionally necessary soon after diagnosis.

Additional tests

Insulin levels are not usually required for therapeutic decision making. A fasting or postprandial C-peptide level (which is indicative of pancreatic insulin production) in type 2 diabetic patients may have some value in predicting response to therapy. As diabetes represents a cardiovascular risk factor, it is often appropriate to check cholesterol and HDL cholesterol (which may be improved to some extent by good diabetes control and diabetic diet).

Summary

Epidemiological evidence indicates that a fasting venous plasma glucose of 7.0 mmol/L is a more sensitive but still reasonably precise threshold for the diagnosis of diabetes than the previous level of 7.8 mmol/L. In most clinical settings, the measurement of a fasting or random glucose will suffice for confirming the diagnosis of diabetes but the OGTT continues to have a significant role in the clinical diagnosis of diabetes mellitus, especially when, despite reasonable suspicion, fasting or random glucose levels are non-diagnostic. The current position statement on the diagnostic criteria as set out by the Australasian Working Party should be adopted while the final WHO recommendation is awaited.

FURTHER READING

Alberti K. G. M. M. and Zimmet P. Z. Definition, diagnosis and classification of diabetes mellitus and its complications. Part 1: diagnosis and classification of diabetes mellitus. Provisional Report of a WHO Consultation. *Diabet Med* 1998; 15: 539–53.

Colman P. G., Thomas D. W., Zimmet P. Z. et al. New classification and criteria for the diagnosis of diabetes mellitus. Position Statement from the Australian Diabetes Society, New Zealand Society for the Study of Diabetes, Royal College of Pathologists of Australasia and Australasian Association of Clinical Biochemists. *Med J Aust* 1999; 170: 375–8.

Expert Committee on the Diagnosis and Classification of Diabetes Mellitus. Report of the Expert Committee on the Diagnosis and Classification of Diabetes Mellitus. *Diabetes Care* 1997; 20: 1183–97.

Diabetes monitoring: use of glycated haemoglobin and glycated protein assays

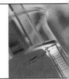

12

G. Jones and D. Chisholm

SYNOPSIS

The measurement of haemoglobin A1c (HbA1c) has emerged over the last decade as the test of choice for monitoring mean glycaemic control in diabetic patients. During this time there has been considerable progress towards standardisation of HbA1c assays to allow comparison of results between different laboratories and different measurement technologies. There remains, however, further work in order to fully characterise the fraction of glycosylated haemoglobin which best reflects recent average blood glucose levels and to ensure high quality testing in all laboratories.

Introduction

The phenomenon of glycation (or glycosylation) of proteins to form neoglycoproteins has long been recognised in the area of food technology as a cause of the 'browning reaction'. In recent years there has been an increasing understanding of the phenomenon of in vivo glycation of proteins, leading to the development of assays which are indicators of mean glycaemic control in patients with diabetes. There has also been intensive study of the possibility that the phenomenon of protein glycation is a significant contributor to long-term diabetic complications—

either by causing changes in structural proteins such as collagen, or by altering function of other proteins such as receptors, enzymes or the apolipoproteins of circulating lipids.

Measurement of circulating neoglycoproteins has now been accepted as a marker of the exposure of circulating proteins to glucose and also of the risk of diabetic complications. Assays of glycated haemoglobin and glycated albumin (fructosamine) are available and each assay reflects the life span of that protein in the circulation; for example, HbA1c indicates glycaemic control over 3 months (the life of the red cell) and fructosamine reflects control over 6 weeks (the life of serum albumin in the circulation). In both cases results are weighted towards recent glycaemic control as recent changes have affected all the protein present at the time of measurement.

Biochemistry of protein glycation

When proteins are exposed to glucose, the carbonyl group of glucose may attach to the ε-amino groups of lysine or the α-amino groups of the N-terminal amino acids of the proteins. This attachment results in the formation of a Schiff base (aldimine) in a reversible reaction. An Amadori rearrangement then results in the non-reversible formation of a ketoamine, after which cyclisation results in the formation of a glycated protein. (See Fig. 12.1.)

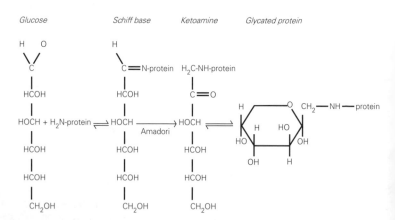

FIGURE 12.1 Glycation of proteins

Glycated proteins are quite stable and are not enzymatically degraded in mammals. Exposure of proteins to high concentrations of glucose over a relatively long period of time may result in the formation of advanced glycosylation end products (AGE) or 'browning'.

Glycation of proteins occurs to some extent in non-diabetic humans at physiological blood glucose levels, so that approximately 1% of serum albumin is normally glycated, as is a small fraction of haemoglobin.

Technical aspects
Haemoglobin A1c

A variety of methods are in routine use for the measurement of glycated haemoglobin. These include ion-exchange chromatography, affinity chromatography, and various immunoassay systems. But each glycated haemoglobin method measures a different glycated component of haemoglobin. Boronate affinity methods separate 'total glycated haemoglobin' according to the structural characteristics of the glycated component. Immunoassay methods also rely on structural differences in haemoglobin species, but they measure only the glycation on the NH_2 terminus of the β-chain (HbA1c specifically). Ion exchange and electrophoretic methods separate HbA1c from other Hb species according to molecular charge. Because of these methodological differences glycated haemoglobin results from different laboratories may vary considerably.[1]

A research goal is to identify the form of glycosylated haemoglobin which best reflects recent average blood glucose concentrations. In practice the current gold standard is the method used to measure HbA1c in the Diabetes Control and Complications Trial (DCCT) which showed a correlation between levels of HbA1c and outcomes in type 1 diabetic patients.[2] A recent U.K. consensus statement has confirmed that HbA1c is the measurement of choice, that methods should be aligned with the DCCT method and that results should be reported as 'DCCT equivalent HbA1c'.[3] The original DCCT method was an in-house HPLC method which is not commercially available; however a U.S. group, the National Glycohaemoglobin Standardisation Program (NGSP), will certify methods and laboratories against this method.[4] Most of the commonly used methods in Australia today are referenced against this standard. This may involve mathematical manipulation of the results; for example, if a method measures total glycated haemoglobin, a factor is used to convert this result to HbA1c. This is not to say that there are no analytical issues of importance in the measurement of HbA1c. Schiff base interference remains an issue in some ion-exchange methods although this is becoming much less common with modern methods. Most immunoassay systems struggle to reach the recommended within-laboratory precision of a coefficient of variation (CV) of less than 3%. The importance of the assay precision can be seen with the example of an assay with CV of 5%. A result from such an assay of 9.0% HbA1c indicates a 95% confidence interval for the result of between 8.1% and 9.9%. Obviously this represents a wide range of possibilities for the state of glycaemic control and also makes detection of significant changes in results difficult. Some variant haemoglobins continue to give grossly different values in some systems.

Despite referencing methods back to the DCCT trial a sample may still give significantly different results when measured in different laboratories. Therefore it is preferable to monitor patients with results from a single laboratory and if differences are seen on changing laboratories they should be discussed with the laboratories concerned before assuming that a change in the patient's glycaemic control has occurred.

Glycated serum proteins

With the rise in understanding and acceptance of HbA1c testing there has been a reduction in the use of other glycated proteins such as fructosamine. The fructosamine assay is largely a measure of glycated albumin and therefore reflects the average blood glucose over the previous 2 to 3 weeks, reflecting the half-life of albumin in the circulation. In general this test is now restricted to circumstances where HbA1c is inappropriate either due to a desire to investigate shorter time intervals or because there is interference with HbA1c measurement.

Clinical use of glycated protein assays

The particular use of the HbA1c (or fructosamine) assay is to provide an index of medium- to long-term control of the diabetes.

This contrasts with the use of self blood glucose monitoring to indicate hour-to-hour or day-to-day changes in control, which may be used to adjust therapy on a daily basis, e.g. in the type 1 patient who may alter insulin doses or carbohydrate intake in response to changes in physical activity.

HbA1c measurements have a particular value in diabetic patients who are unwilling or unable to do regular fingerprick blood glucose measurements, or in situations where there may be a doubt as to the validity of the fingerprick blood glucose measurements, such as a faulty monitoring device. Patients attending a physician or clinic may be affected by stress or altered lifestyle routine on that day and have higher than usual blood glucose measurements ('white coat hyperglycaemia')—a satisfactory HbA1c level on these occasions is very reassuring.

Although HbA1c levels correspond to initiation and progression of diabetic complications (especially microvascular disease) physicians need to be realistic in setting target goals. Even with the intense supervision and aggressive therapy in the DCCT few patients with type 1 diabetes achieved a normal HbA1c and the mean of the intensively treated group was approximately 7.0%—about 15% above the upper limit of normal. Even at this level of control there was a three-fold increase in hypoglycaemic reactions and a similar proportionate increase in severe hypoglycaemic reactions. Most diabetologists would feel happy if type 1 diabetic patients could achieve HbA1c levels around the 7% to 7.5% range. In patients with hypoglycaemia unawareness and problems with severe hypoglycaemic reactions the target HbA1c may need to be even a little higher.

In type 2 diabetic patients who are less susceptible to hypoglycaemia, and especially in those on low levels of medication, it is desirable and often possible to achieve HbA1c levels in the 6% to 7% range. However the United Kingdom Prospective Diabetes Study clearly demonstrated the difficulty in maintaining this control over the long term with presently available therapy, and the need to aggressively add further medication when a satisfactory HbA1c level is not achieved.

Although HbA1c levels are closely correlated with the development or progression of microvascular disease and neuropathy, the relationship with cardiovascular events and mortality is less impressive and a number of studies indicate that attention to blood pressure and lipid control has great importance with regard to cardiovascular outcome.

It should be mentioned that in situations of more rapid turnover (e.g. some anaemias for HbA1c or proteinuria for fructosamine) the glycated protein result may be lower than expected for the degree of glycaemia due to shorter exposure of the protein to the prevailing glucose level.

In the chronic stable situation, the performance of a glycosylated haemoglobin or serum protein assay at 3–6 month intervals would be considered reasonable by most physicians expert in diabetes management.

Glycated protein assays have not proved suitable for the diagnosis, or exclusion of the diagnosis, of diabetes mellitus or impaired glucose tolerance. However as an index of metabolic control in individual patients, glycated protein assays have great importance in research studies assessing the relationship of glycaemic control to the progression of complications or other outcome measures; they may also be used as important parameters for audit of outcome for clinic populations.

REFERENCES

1 Little R. R. Recent progress in glycohemoglobin (HbA1c) testing. *Diabetes Care* 2000; 23: 265.

2 The Diabetes Control and Complications Trial Research Group: The effect of intensive treatment of diabetes on the development and progression of long-term complications in insulin-dependent diabetes mellitus. *N Engl J Med* 1993; 329: 977–86.

3 Marshall S. M. and Barth J. H. Standardization of HbA1c measurements: a consensus statement. *Ann Clin Biochem* 2000; 37: 45–6.

4 National Glycohemoglobin Standardisation Program. University of Missouri, http://www.missouri.edu/~diabetes/ngsp.html

Tests of thyroid function

13

J. R. Stockigt

Introduction

The diversity of clinical presentation of both thyrotoxicosis and hypothyroidism makes it difficult to rule out these conditions on clinical grounds alone. Studies of unselected patients assessed by primary care physicians show that clinical acumen alone lacks sensitivity and specificity in detecting previously undiagnosed thyroid dysfunction.[1] In up to one-third of patients evaluated for suspected thyroid disease by specialists, laboratory results lead to revision of the clinical assessment.[2]

Laboratory tests facilitate early diagnosis of thyroid dysfunction before clinical features are obvious, but increased diagnostic sensitivity carries the price of decreased specificity. It is not easy to distinguish erroneous results from those that indicate subclinical dysfunction.

Who should be tested?

While there is little doubt that serum TSH should be measured whenever an abnormality of thyroid function is suspected, there are three patient groups in whom routine testing is appropriate. Neonatal screening for congenital hypothyroidism is now widely established. Recent recommendations endorsed by the American

College of Physicians[3] suggest that thyroid dysfunction is sufficiently common in women over 50 to justify routine testing in this group when they present for medical care (case-finding); the majority of abnormal findings will identify subclinical rather than overt dysfunction (see below). Further, the finding of slight intellectual impairment in the offspring of women who were even mildly hypothyroid during pregnancy[4] may be an indication for testing of thyroid function, either before conception, or as early as possible in pregnancy. Recent American Thyroid Association guidelines extend these indications to recommend that all adults have their serum TSH concentrations measured, beginning at age 35 and every 5 years thereafter.[5] Evidence for the benefit of this approach in males is so far lacking.

Technical aspects

All current methods of measuring TSH, T_4 and T_3 in serum, whether by immunoassay or immunometric techniques, are comparative—they depend on the assumption that the unknown sample and the assay standards are identical in all measurable characteristics other than the concentration of analyte. When this condition is not fulfilled, for example when the sample shows anomalous binding of tracer to serum proteins or antibodies, the assay result will be spurious.[6]

Measurement of serum TSH

Secretion of TSH from the anterior pituitary is regulated by negative feedback from the serum free T_4 and free T_3 concentrations. The serum TSH response to changes in serum free T_4 is logarithmic; a two-fold change in free T_4 induces an approximate 10-fold change in TSH. Reference values for serum immunoreactive TSH are generally in the range 0.3–4 mU/L (Table 13.1), but the geometric mean and median values are at about 1.0 mU/L, an important fact in selecting the TSH target value during replacement therapy.

Immunometric TSH assays that use two antibodies against different epitopes of TSH have greatly improved assay sensitivity. Serum TSH can now be precisely measured to at least 0.03 mU/L, so that the lowest concentrations in normal subjects are clearly distinguishable from those found in thyrotoxicosis, provided assay

TABLE 13.1 Human reference ranges for serum thyroid hormones and TSH*

HORMONE	REFERENCE RANGE
Thyroxine, total (T_4)	60–140 nmol/L
Free T_4	10–25 pmol/L†
Triiodothyronine, total (T_3)	1.1–2.7 nmol/L‡
Free T_3	3–8 pmol/L†‡
TSH	0.3–4.0 mU/L

* These ranges should be determined for the particular methods used in each laboratory.
† Variable, depending on the details of method
‡ Higher values in childhood[7]

sensitivity remains optimal. However, assay specificity is not perfect, and false-positive detectable serum TSH is still found in occasional patients with definite thyrotoxicosis. (This artefact is more common than TSH-producing pituitary tumour.) Subnormal but detectable TSH values do not usually indicate thyrotoxicosis, although values in the range 0.03–0.4 mU/L are common in patients with goitre who merit follow-up because they may later develop thyrotoxicosis. During severe illness, serum TSH is often subnormal without indicating any persistent abnormality of thyroid function; transient increases to above normal may occur during the recovery phase.

Measurement of serum T_4 and T_3

Concentrations of total serum T_4 and T_3 reflect not only hormone production, but also the number and affinity of plasma protein-binding sites. Total concentrations vary in direct relationship to protein binding, while serum free T_4 and free T_3 concentrations should not, if measured by valid methods. Reference ranges are shown in Table 13.1. Serum total and free T_3 concentrations are somewhat higher in children.

There have been many approaches to the assay of serum free T_4 and free T_3 concentrations; the validity of some methods is questionable and no current method actually measures the free hormone concentration in undisturbed, undiluted serum in a way that reflects in vivo conditions.[6] Circulating drugs that inhibit protein binding generally lead to an underestimate of free T_4. Initial evaluation of new serum free T_4 methods has often been incomplete and interference may be noted only after a technique has been used for some time, as in the effect of abnormal albumin binding of T_4, rheumatoid factor or heparin to produce spuriously high serum free T_4 estimates.[6]

Serum T_3 should also be measured in suspected or treated thyrotoxicosis when serum T_4 is normal and serum TSH is suppressed. Serum T_3 is important in the diagnosis of amiodarone-induced thyrotoxicosis, which should not be based on T_4 excess alone. Serum T_3 establishes the extent of hormone excess during suppressive therapy with T_4, or when an intentional T_4 overdose has been taken. Serum T_3 has no place in the diagnosis of hypothyroidism and, because of its short plasma half-life, is not useful in assessing replacement with T_3.

The TSH–T_4 relationship

Whatever strategy is used for first-line testing, a sensitive serum TSH assay and a valid serum free T_4 estimate are necessary for *definitive* assessment of thyroid status. The assumptions that are fundamental to the diagnostic value of this relationship have been considered in detail.[6] When both parameters are considered together, specificity is excellent, because there is no known clinical or laboratory artefact that can cause the characteristic diagonal deviations that define true thyroid dysfunction. The large difference between the half-lives of TSH (1 hour) and T_4 (1 week) accounts for many transient anomalies in this T_4–TSH relationship if the sample has been taken under non-steady-state conditions.

TSH as the initial test of thyroid function

A general algorithm for the assessment of thyroid function based on initial measurement of TSH is shown in Figure 13.2. With current TSH assays, the reference interval for euthyroid subjects is clearly separate from values typical of thyrotoxicosis. Abnormal TSH values lead to further assays as shown. Serum TSH may give an incomplete or inaccurate assessment of thyroid status. Assay of free T_4 is required in the presence of a normal serum TSH if pituitary dysfunction is suspected, during the early treatment of thyroid dysfunction and during critical illness.

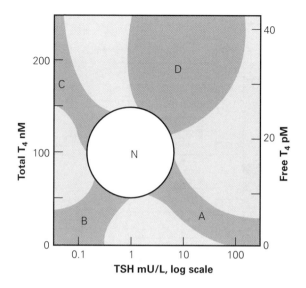

Sampling in steady conditions
Undisturbed tropic–target gland relationship
No major effect of unmeasured active hormones
Tissue responses reflect hormone concentration
Appropriate reference ranges
Adequate assay sensitivity in subnormal range

FIGURE 13.1

The common types of thyroid dysfunction are defined by characteristic diagonal deviations from the normal T_4–TSH relationship that result from negative feedback between target gland and trophic hormones.[6] Figure 13.1 shows primary hypothyroidism due to target gland failure (A), failure of TSH secretion (B), autonomous or abnormally stimulated target gland function (C), and primary excess of TSH or thyroid hormone resistance (D). Abnormal results that fall outside these areas suggest that some other factor has disturbed this relationship, or that the sample has been collected under non-steady-state conditions. The assumptions that underlie the diagnostic use of the trophic hormone–target gland relationship are listed below the figure.

In the absence of associated disease, a normal serum TSH concentration has over 99% negative predictive value in ruling out primary hypothyroidism and thyrotoxicosis. Assessment of untreated subjects now commonly begins with measurement of TSH alone, with T_4 and T_3 assays added only if TSH is abnormal,

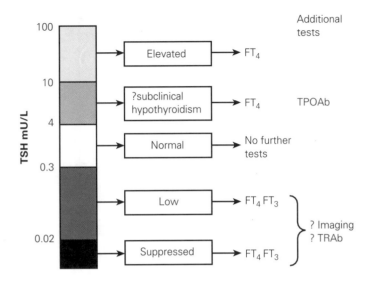

FIGURE 13.2 Protocol for the assessment of thyroid function based on initial assay of serum TSH

(Reproduced with permission from *Oxford Textbook of Endocrinology*, 2001, in press)

or if an abnormality of TSH secretion is suspected. When serum TSH is elevated, free T_4 must be measured to distinguish between overt and subclinical hypothyroidism, while a suppressed TSH level should be followed by assay of both free T_4 and free T_3 to distinguish subclinical from overt thyrotoxicosis and to identify T_3 toxicosis.

The use of serum TSH as the sole initial test of thyroid function may lead to incorrect or incomplete assessment of thyroid status:

■ when pituitary function is abnormal

■ during the first months of treatment for thyrotoxicosis or hypothyroidism, when TSH normalisation may lag behind changes in T_4 and T_3 and clinical response

■ during an associated illness, particularly related to the effects of medications.

Concordant results

When clinical and laboratory findings are concordant with clinical features, two important questions should be asked: how severe is the disorder, and what is the cause of the abnormality?

How severe is the disorder?

Assessment of severity is a judgement based on clinical rather than laboratory findings, because the latter give no indication of duration of exposure. Proximal myopathy or heart failure are markers of severe thyrotoxicosis, while drowsiness, bradycardia and marked slowing of reflex relaxation indicate severe hypothyroidism.

What is the cause of the abnormality?

Abnormal hormone levels, associated with a clinical picture of thyroid dysfunction, do not establish the causal abnormality. When overactivity is diagnosed, the choice of treatment will be different for Graves' disease, subacute thyroiditis, excessive hormone ingestion, solitary toxic adenoma, toxic multinodular goitre and transient postpartum thyrotoxicosis.

Discordant results

When there is discordance between laboratory results and clinical findings, a distinction needs to be made between anomalous assay results due to specific or non-specific assay interference and findings that indicate previously unsuspected or subclinical disease. Consideration of the fundamental assumptions that underlie the diagnostic use of the TSH–T_4 relationship (Fig. 13.1) may give a clue to the discrepancy. When clinical and laboratory findings are discordant, clinical reassessment should be followed by consideration of four questions: why was the test done, what was the timing of the sample, is drug therapy or an associated illness involved, and are other family members affected?

Why was the test done?

If a result is normal when done to confirm a fairly confident clinical diagnosis, a repeat sample should be taken with a request for second-line assays, e.g. T_3 measurement in suspected thyrotoxicosis. When an abnormality is reported in response to a test done with a low index of suspicion, clinical reassessment should precede treatment.

Timing of the sample

When testing to monitor therapy, duration of treatment should be considered to confirm that a steady state has been reached. Clinical features can lag several weeks behind changes in hormone level. Important causes of non-steady-state findings include subacute thyroiditis, recovery from severe illness, postpartum thyroid dysfunction, acute psychiatric illness, and sampling early in the course of T_4 replacement or antithyroid drug therapy, or in the first 2–3 months after thyroid surgery or treatment with [131]I.

Could drug therapy or an associated illness account for an anomaly?

Many drugs can alter thyroid hormone levels by the mechanisms listed in Table 13.2. Some drugs have complex multiple actions. The most difficult is amiodarone, which has multiple effects related to iodine excess, inhibition of T_3 formation from T_4 and a unique form of severe persistent thyroiditis that results in uncontrolled T_4 and T_3 release. Severe illness is associated with many drug-related changes that can make interpretation of routine tests extremely difficult.[8]

Are other family members affected?

If an abnormality is identified that causes misleading results by commonly used assay techniques, it may be appropriate to identify affected family members who are also at risk of misdiagnosis.

Subclinical disease

The more widespread the testing of thyroid function, the greater the proportion of results in which only TSH is outside the reference range. The clinical importance of subclinical thyroid dysfunction is summarised in Table 13.3 (on page 78). A TSH level that is double the upper normal limit is no immediate cause for concern, although it predicts the probable later development of overt hypothyroidism. During the gradual progression of thyroid

TABLE 13.2 Medications that influence thyroid hormone or TSH levels*

Inhibit TSH secretion	Dopaminergics, glucocorticoids
Deliver iodine load†	Radiologic contrast agents, amiodarone, topical preparations
Inhibit thyroid hormone release	Lithium, glucocorticoids
Inhibit T_4–T_3 conversion	Amiodarone, glucocorticoids, beta blockers‡
Inhibit binding of T_4 and T_3 to plasma proteins	Furosemide, salicylates, non-steroidal anti-inflammatory agents‡, phenytoin, carbamazepine, heparin§
Increase concentration of T_4-binding globulin	Oestrogen, heroin, methadone, clofibrate, 5-fluorouracil, tamoxifen, glucocorticoids
Increase clearance of iodothyronines	Barbiturates, phenytoin, carbamazepine, rifampicin, sertraline?, fluoxetine?, dothiepin?
Impair absorption of ingested T_4	Aluminium hydroxide, ferrous sulfate, cholestyramine, colestipol, sucralfate, soya preparations, calcium carbonate
Modify thyroid hormone action (?)	Amiodarone, phenytoin

* Conventional antithyroid drugs excluded
† Effect depends on thyroid status
‡ Some members of the group
§ In vitro effect of in vivo heparin administration[9]

dysfunction, TSH may become abnormal months or years before there is a diagnostic change in the serum concentrations of T_4 or T_3. Clinical follow-up with retesting every 6–12 months may be preferred to immediate treatment.

Integration of tests of thyroid function with other investigations

When thyroid function is abnormal, additional diagnostic information can be gained from antibody studies, imaging techniques and measurement of thyroglobulin. The investigation of thyroid masses per se is not considered here.

TABLE 13.3 Importance of subclinical thyroid dysfunction

SUBCLINICAL THYROTOXICOSIS (SUPPRESSED TSH, NORMAL FREE T_4, FREE T_3)
Progression to overt thyrotoxicosis
Exposure to iodine may precipitate severe thyrotoxicosis
Three-fold increased risk of atrial fibrillation[10]
Osteoporosis risk may be increased

SUBCLINICAL HYPOTHYROIDISM (INCREASED TSH, NORMAL FREE T_4)
Non-specific symptoms may improve with treatment[11]
Progression to overt hypothyroidism (? 5% per year)
Adverse effect on foetal brain development in pregnancy[4]
Independent risk factor for coronary disease?[12]
Beneficial effect of treatment on lipids?[13]

Antibody measurements

In subclinical hypothyroidism, the presence of thyroid peroxidase (TPO) antibodies indicates a four-to-five-fold increase in the chance of developing overt hypothyroidism.[14] The finding of persistently positive thyrotropin receptor antibody (TRAb) is useful in indicating that apparent remission of Graves' disease is unlikely to be sustained. TRAb measurement can indicate the possibility of neonatal thyrotoxicosis in the infant of a mother with autoimmune thyroid disease and may also define the aetiology of atypical eye disease.

Thyroid imaging

The finding of negligible technetium uptake can be a key feature in confirming that thyrotoxicosis is due to thyroiditis, iodine contamination or factitious ingestion of thyroid hormone. Imaging also can confirm a 'hot' nodule as the predominant source of thyroid hormone excess. Computerised tomography is valuable in identifying the extent of retrosternal extension, but contrast agents must be avoided. Colour-flow Doppler has been reported to differentiate between type 1 and type 2 amiodarone-induced thyrotoxicosis.[15]

Thyroglobulin

In the follow-up of differentiated thyroid cancer, an undetectable serum thyroglobulin concentration in the presence of high serum TSH indicates effective ablation. Thyroglobulin is undetectable in thyrotoxicosis factitia, and generally extremely high in subacute thyroiditis and in amiodarone-induced thyrotoxicosis.

Indices of thyroid hormone action

While there is currently no diagnostically reliable laboratory index of peripheral thyroid hormone action, some tests including sex-steroid-binding globulin, serum ferritin, serum angiotensin converting enzyme, as well as measurement of oxygen consumption, systolic time interval and ultrasonographic parameters of cardiac contractility, may be useful in following an individual's response in situations of suspected thyroid hormone resistance, or during long-term suppressive therapy with T_4.

Summary

A normal serum TSH value has a high negative predictive value in ruling out primary thyroid dysfunction; if TSH is abnormal, serum free T_4 (and serum T_3 if TSH is suppressed) is required to identify overt thyroid dysfunction. Diagnosis is based on characteristic changes in the trophic hormone–target gland relationship. Clinical reassessment, followed if necessary by repeat measurement, is the first step in the evaluation of clinically discordant results, which are more often due to sampling under non-steady-state conditions than to assay inaccuracy or a rare disease. Widespread testing of thyroid function identifies more subclinical dysfunction (abnormal TSH, normal T_4 and T_3), than overt disease. Effective long-term management of overt or subclinical thyroid disease depends on follow-up, which in turn requires education of both patients and practitioners.

REFERENCES

1 Eggertsen R., Petersen K., Lundberg P. A. et al. Screening for thyroid disease in a primary care unit with thyroid stimulating hormone assay with low detection limit. *Br Med J* 1988; 297: 1586–92.

2 Jarlov A. E., Nygaard B., Hegedus L. et al. Observer variation in the clinical and laboratory evaluation of patients with thyroid dysfunction and goiter. *Thyroid* 1998; 8(5): 393–8.

3 Helfand M. and Redfern C. C. Screening for thyroid disease: an update. *Ann Intern Med* 1998; 129: 144–58.

4 Haddow J. E., Palomaki G. E., Allan W. C. et al. Maternal thyroid deficiency during pregnancy and subsequent neuropsychological development of the child. *N Engl J Med* 1999; 341: 549–55.

5 Ladenson P. W., Singer P. A., Ain K. B. et al. American Thyroid Association guidelines for detection of thyroid dysfunction. *Arch Intern Med* 2000; 160: 1573–5.

6 Stockigt J. R. Serum TSH and thyroid hormone measurements and assessment of thyroid hormone transport. In: Braverman L. E. and Utiger R. G., eds. *Werner and Ingbar's The Thyroid*. 8th edn. Philadelphia: Lippincott, Williams & Wilkins, 2000, pp. 376–92.

7 Verheecke P. Free triiodothyronine concentration in serum of 1050 euthyroid children is inversely related to their age. *Clin Chem* 1997; 43: 963–7.

8 Stockigt J. R. Guidelines for diagnosis and monitoring of thyroid disease: nonthyroidal illness. *Clin Chem* 1996; 42: 188–92.

9 Mendel C. M., Frost P. H., Kunitake S. T. and Cavalieri R. R. Mechanism of the heparin-induced increase in the concentration of free thyroxine in plasma. *J Clin Endocrinol Metab* 1987; 65: 1259–64.

10 Sawin C. T., Geller A., Wolf P. A., et al. Low serum thyrotropin concentrations as a risk factor for arterial fibrillation in older persons. *N Engl J Med* 1994; 331: 1249–52.

11 Nystrom E., Caidahl K., Fager G. et al. A double-blind cross-over 12 month study of l-thyroxine treatment of women with subclinical hypothyroidism. *Clin Endocrinol* 1988; 29: 63–76.

12 Hak A. E., Pols H. A. P., Visser T. J. et al. Subclinical hypothyroidism is an independent risk factor for atherosclerosis and myocardial infarction in elderly women: The Rotterdam Study. *Ann Int Med* 2000; 132: 270–8.

13 Diekman T., Lansberg P. J., Kastelstein J. J. P. et al. Prevalence and correction of hypothyroidism in a large cohort of patients with dyslipidemia. *Arch Int Med* 1995; 155: 1490–5.

14 Vanderpump M. P. J., Tunbridge W. M. G., French J. M. et al. The incidence of thyroid disorders in the community: a twenty-year follow-up of the Whickham Survey. *Clin Endocrinol* 1995; 43: 55–68.

15 Bogazzi F. et al. Color flow Doppler sonography rapidly differentiates Type I and Type II amiodarone-induced thyrotoxicosis. *Thyroid* 1997; 7: 541–5.

Interpretation of arterial blood gases

14

L.G. Olson

SYNOPSIS

Arterial blood gas measurements have become a core element in the initial evaluation of acutely ill patients. Much of this use is inappropriate and, in particular, use of blood gas measurements to assess tissue oxygenation is inappropriate. Interpretation of arterial blood gases requires understanding of two physiological principles: (1) alveolar and therefore arterial PCO_2 is inversely related to alveolar ventilation (as ventilation halves PCO_2 doubles), and (2) all hypoxaemia is due either to a rise in alveolar PCO_2 or to abnormal ventilation/perfusion (V/Q) ratios in the lung. The most important corollary of the first principle is that marked rises in PCO_2 are late developments in lung disease, and to wait for them to occur is usually to wait too long. The most important corollary of the second principle is that all lung diseases cause hypoxaemia by the same mechanism and that this mechanism is not closely connected with the pathological processes, and that therefore arterial PO_2 is not usually helpful either diagnostically or in assessing disease severity.

Introduction

Arterial blood gas measurement is a relatively recent development. Arterial pH and PCO_2 were first measured for patient care in the early 1950s, and PO_2 in the early 1960s. The process of measuring blood gases turned out to be easy to automate, and robust, simple and inexpensive machines have made blood gas analysis very widely available. This, and the illusion that arterial blood gases represent a window into the function of the lung, has led to overuse of blood gases, and over-interpretation of the results. Measuring arterial PO_2, in particular, commonly receives attention quite disproportionate to its utility.

Technical aspects

The first matter to be considered is units of measurement. The most widely used unit is the millimetre of mercury (mmHg), an unfortunate choice because mmHg is not a unit of pressure at all. The torr (for Torricelli) is a non-SI unit of pressure; for practical purposes 1 torr = 1 mmHg. The most correct unit of measurement of pressure is the kPa, but, as in the case of blood pressure, there has been very little progress towards replacing mmHg with kPa. Millimetres of mercury can be (and should be, but will not be in this chapter) converted to kPa by dividing by 7.5.

There are two ways in which inattention to technical aspects of blood gas sampling and measurement can cause problems: the measurement can be inaccurate and the measurement can be misleading.

An inaccurate measurement means that the measured values are not the ones the blood had when it was in the patient. Machine error—the values on the printout are not the ones in the blood in the machine—is rare with modern machines if they are carefully maintained. Inaccurate results can occur (1) if there are air bubbles in the sample, (2) if analysis is delayed, so that metabolism by cellular elements in the blood depletes oxygen and adds carbon dioxide, and (3), most importantly, if the temperature of analysis is not the same as the patient's temperature. Analyses are conducted at 37°C unless the machine is reset to a different temperature, and if the patient's temperature is higher than 37°C the measured PO_2 and PCO_2 are lower than the real values. Conversely, if the patient is hypothermic the measured values of PO_2 and PCO_2 are higher than the real values. For PO_2 the error increases as the saturation of haemoglobin with oxygen falls, and reaches 7.5% per degree Celsius when S_aO_2 is less than 90%. For PCO_2 the error is less: the measured value differs from the real value by about 5% per degree

Celsius that the patient's temperature differs from 37°C, and the error does not depend on S_aO_2.

Misleading values of arterial blood gases arise most often from failure to ensure steady-state conditions (conditions in which the excretion of CO_2 from the lungs is equal to the metabolic production of CO_2) . If a patient hyperventilates in response to a painful needle-stick the output of CO_2 from the lungs exceeds metabolic production of CO_2, and the PCO_2 in the blood does not reflect body CO_2 content. Another common cause of sampling under non-steady-state conditions is underestimating the time it takes for changes in inspired oxygen levels to affect alveolar gas and therefore arterial blood. In patients with lung disease poorly ventilated areas of the lung will take 30 minutes (and some alveoli will take even longer in severe airway disease) to equilibrate with the gas entering the airway, and therefore the arterial PO_2 will take the same extended time to reflect fully changes in inspired gas composition.

How long it takes changes in a patient's clinical state to be reflected in blood gas tensions is discussed below.

Physiological aspects

The key physiological fact about blood gases is that the central parameters (PO_2 and PCO_2) reflect aspects of the body's function which are, in a clinical context, largely independent. Oxygen levels reflect the gas exchange function of the lung, and carbon dioxide levels reflect the mechanical function of the chest wall and its muscles.

Oxygen

PO_2 reflects the gas exchanging function of the lung. This function is determined, for practical purposes, by the distribution of ventilation and perfusion to each area of the lung (the 'V/Q ratio'). It is unusual for there to be any failure of diffusion across the alveolar-capillary membrane (that is, gas tensions in an alveolus and in the capillary blood leaving that alveolus are nearly always identical). It is important that it is the V/Q *ratio* that determines gas exchange: it is often forgotten that a doubling of perfusion without a rise in ventilation will cause hypoxaemia just as readily as a halving of ventilation without a fall in perfusion.

Hypoxaemia is caused by areas of the lung with low V/Q ratios (roughly, less than 1). The lower the V/Q ratio in an area of the lung the more marked the hypoxaemia in the blood leaving that area of the lung, and the lower the final PO_2 when all the blood is mixed together in the systemic arterial circulation. There is no way, however, to tell from the arterial blood gases whether there are large areas of lung with mildly abnormal V/Q ratios or small areas with severely abnormal ratios, or even a right-to-left shunt entirely outside the lung.

The distribution of V/Q ratios in the lung is disrupted readily. Arterial PO_2 therefore falls early, even in mild disorders, and in both lung and chest wall disorders. That is, hypoxaemia is very sensitive for lung and chest wall disease but highly non-specific. In particular, painful chest wall conditions are associated with a surprising degree of hypoxaemia, and blood gas analysis is not an appropriate way to look for the presence of lung disease in a patient with chest pain or breathlessness.

A second important physiological point which impairs the utility of measuring PO_2 is that tissue oxygen uptake has little relation to arterial PO_2. If the circulation is intact oxygen uptake is constant across a very wide range of PO_2, and even marked hypoxaemia need not imply any degree of tissue anoxia. The caveat that the circulation must be intact is important, and delivery-dependent oxygen uptake has been observed in patients with acute critical illness, but if information on tissue oxygenation is wanted it is in organ function, not in arterial blood gas tensions, that it must be looked for.

It is also important that body stores of oxygen are small. They consist mainly of the oxygen bound to haemoglobin and myoglobin, and the oxygen in the air in the lung. Because these stores are small in relation to consumption they are rapidly consumed when replacement stops. Arterial PO_2 therefore falls very quickly—1–2 mmHg a second—when breathing stops.

Carbon dioxide

Arterial PCO_2 is inversely proportional to alveolar ventilation (that is, as alveolar ventilation halves, PCO_2 doubles—see Fig. 14.1). Alveolar ventilation is not the same as ventilation in and out of the mouth, but discussing the difference is beyond the scope of this chapter. Arterial PCO_2 also depends on the body's production of CO_2, and this is more variable than is commonly realised. Fever and muscle contraction increase CO_2 production markedly, and conversely muscle paralysis reduces it. Normally, ventilation is driven by changes in CO_2, and (for example) exercise is associated with a seamless increase in ventilation so that it is precisely isocapnic. This mechanism is lost if ventilation is fixed or limited, and changes in arterial PCO_2 cannot be interpreted without considering the possibility of changes in CO_2 production. Because PCO_2 is inversely proportional to ventilation, if PCO_2 is initially low ventilation will fall a lot before PCO_2 rises a lot. For example, if PCO_2 starts at 20 mmHg ventilation must fall from 10 L/min to 5 L/min before PCO_2 reaches 40 mmHg, but a further fall of only 2.5 L/min will cause PCO_2 to rise to 80 mmHg. This has two important corollaries: once the PCO_2 is above normal most of the possible decline in ventilation has already occurred, and when the PCO_2 is high clinically insignificant changes in ventilation can produce quite large changes in PCO_2.

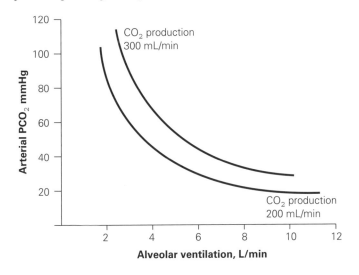

FIGURE 14.1 Reltionship between alveolar ventilation and arterial PCO_2 at two levels of metabolic CO_2 production

Because PCO_2 primarily reflects ventilation it is primarily a measure of the ventilatory pump. Gas exchange disturbances (abnormal V/Q ratios) have little impact on PCO_2. That is, if the

PCO_2 is high it is because the patient is not breathing enough, not because of a problem with gas exchange. Not breathing can be because the patient *can't breathe* or because they *won't breathe*. *Can't breathe* means usually that the respiratory muscles are not strong enough to move air given the resistance to air flow (as in acute severe asthma), and the problem can be either that the load is overwhelming or that the muscles are weak or fatigued. Occasionally *can't breathe* means that the muscles are mechanically disadvantaged, as by a flail chest. *Won't breathe* means malfunction of the respiratory control system (for example, by administration of a narcotic). Usually it is fairly easy to tell 'can't' from 'won't', although coexistent problems of both types (e.g. a postoperative patient with COAD whose muscles are inhibited by abdominal pain and who is given narcotic analgesia) are common.

An important physiological point in interpreting PCO_2 is that the size of body CO_2 stores is very large (15–20 L), so that the 200–300 mL of CO_2 added each minute by metabolism do not make a large difference. In steady-state conditions arterial PCO_2 measures body CO_2 stores, and therefore arterial PCO_2 rises quite slowly when ventilation is inadequate (in contrast to the rate of fall of PO_2). During apnoea PCO_2 rises abruptly to the mixed venous level (about 46 mmHg) but thereafter only 3–5 mmHg a minute—as long as catastrophic falls in PO_2 are prevented. This means, first of all, that a very high arterial PCO_2 implies a prolonged deficiency of ventilation, and conversely that PCO_2 will fall only slowly when that deficiency is reversed, and secondly that if PCO_2 is very high gas exchange cannot be very bad, because otherwise the fall in PO_2 would have been fatal.

Is the result abnormal, and what action is needed if it is?
Oxygen

As noted above, arterial PO_2 is readily perturbed, and the changes in the lung with ageing cause a fall in PO_2. As a rule of thumb predicted PO_2 is 100 mmHg minus (age/4), so an 80 year old has a predicted PO_2 of 80 mmHg. If there is hypoxaemia either there is inadequate ventilation (in which case PCO_2 will be high) or there is an abnormal distribution of V/Q ratios. All lung disease does this, and diagnostically hypoxaemia rarely means anything other than that there is some sort of lung disease. Therapeutically, a high PO_2

does not mean there is adequate tissue oxygenation and a low PO_2 is not, in itself, a reason to provide supplementary oxygen.

Arterial PO_2 is reduced if PCO_2 is high because CO_2 occupies space in the alveoli and reduces the alveolar PO_2. The distinction between a PO_2 low because of a high PCO_2 and one low because of gas exchange abnormality requires calculation of the alveolar-arterial oxygen difference (A-a DO_2). It is important that this is a mean difference for the lung as a whole, and does not imply any difference between alveolar and capillary oxygen tensions (which, as noted above, is uncommon). As a rule of thumb, *in a patient breathing room air* the A-a DO_2 is equal to 150 minus the sum of the arterial PCO_2 and the arterial PCO_2. The A-a DO_2 is about 10 mmHg in young people and rises with age (predicted A-a DO_2 is 10 + (age/4)). The A-a DO_2 provides no more or different information than the PO_2 unless PCO_2 is high.

If the patient is not breathing room air the alveolar air equation must be used to calculate alveolar PCO_2 and thus A-a DO_2. There are two traps here. The first is that unless the patient is breathing room air or through a cuffed endotracheal tube attached to a sealed oxygen source the inspired PO_2 cannot be estimated, and the A-a DO_2 cannot be calculated, even approximately. The temptation to calculate A-a DO_2 for patients on Venturi masks and nasal cannulas must be resisted! The second is that, because it may take a long time for alveolar gas to reflect changes in inspired gas composition one cannot remove supplementary oxygen, take a blood gas sample immediately, and calculate the A-a DO_2. Generally, it is necessary to wait at least 20 minutes after removing supplementary oxygen before a patient can be taken to be breathing room air.

As noted above, a low PO_2 is very sensitive for the presence of disease, but very non-specific. An important case of this is the patient suspected of pulmonary embolic disease. The great majority of patients with pulmonary embolism have a low PO_2 — but so do the great majority of patients with a similar clinical picture but no pulmonary embolism (Fig. 14.2).

Carbon dioxide

Arterial PCO_2 is normally about 40 mmHg, but because ventilation is liable to increase for clinically uninteresting reasons such as anxiety low values are of little importance except in an

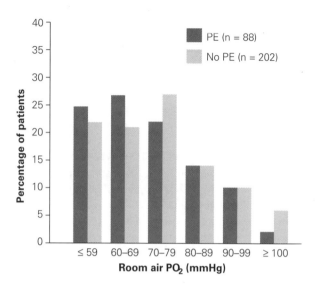

FIGURE 14.2 Arterial PO₂ in patients with pulmonary embolism on pulmonary angiography (filled columns) and in patients suspected of pulmonary embolism but with normal pulmonary angiograms

From Stien P. D., Terrin M. L., Hales C. A. et al. Clinical, laboratory, roentgenographic, and electrocardiographic findings in patients with acute pulmonary embolism and no pre-existing cardiac or pulmonary disease. *Chest* 1991; 100: 598–603.

acid-base context. The possibility of high values, on the other hand, is the fundamental reason arterial blood gases are done.

As noted above, high values reflect advanced disease of the respiratory pump, and often indicate imminent disaster. The respiratory pump has a large reserve capacity, and normally adapts with exquisite precision to changes in CO_2 production. Even a small rise in PCO_2 therefore represents severe disease of the chest wall or respiratory muscles. That is, elevated PCO_2 is insensitive for disease of the respiratory pump, but highly specific. Because of the relationship between ventilation and PCO_2 shown in Figure 14.1 a patient with rib fractures and a PCO_2 of 45 mmHg is in danger of catastrophic respiratory failure: a PCO_2 of 60 mmHg would not be much worse news. When respiratory muscle weakness (as in Guillain-Barré syndrome) is the problem it is the vital capacity (not the FEV_1!) that should be monitored, not the arterial PCO_2. To wait for the PCO_2 to rise is to wait far too long.

Plasma urea

15

T. H. Mathew

SYNOPSIS

Plasma urea is an end product of protein catabolism and, because it is mainly excreted by the kidney and is easily measured, became a popular way to measure renal function. However, because the plasma concentration of urea is subject to many extrarenal variables it has been replaced by plasma creatinine as the mainstay for day-to-day assessment of renal function. Plasma urea remains a useful tool in clinical management when used with insight for it provides information not only about renal function but about the state of hydration, protein catabolic rate and nutritional status.

Introduction

A generation ago plasma urea (then called blood urea as the estimation was performed on whole blood), which is quick and simple to measure by hand, was the standard measure used clinically to estimate renal function on a day-by-day basis. The plasma urea concentration, however, depends on urine flow and is affected by the highly variable production rate (see below), making it an unsatisfactory tool for renal function assessment. These same factors mean that urea clearance is never used alone these days as a means of assessing glomerular filtration rate. Urea clearance does have a use in one setting. In patients with marked renal dysfunction (e.g. when the plasma creatinine > 400 μmol/L) the urea clearance significantly underestimates the glomerular filtration rate. At this same level of renal function the creatinine clearance significantly overestimates the true glomerular filtration rate. It has been shown that a simple and accurate estimate of the glomerular filtration rate in this situation can be achieved by taking the mean of the urea and the creatinine clearances. This calculation has been accepted in the draft Australian guidelines (CARI) as the best means of determining glomerular filtration rate in the assessment of the need for initiation of dialysis.

Technical aspects

Confusion may arise when the plasma urea is expressed as plasma urea nitrogen (BUN). This means of expressing the plasma urea, although widespread in North America, is rarely used in Australia. There is no advantage in expressing plasma urea as BUN. It is sufficient to be aware that 1 gram molecular weight of urea (equals 60 g) contains 2 atomic weights of nitrogen (equals 28 g). Accordingly the factor for converting urea mass units to those of urea nitrogen is 0.47, and for converting urea nitrogen to urea mass units the conversion factor is 2.1.

Urea is readily diffusible through most of the body tissues including red blood cells. Accordingly, the intracellular level is the same as that found in plasma and as a consequence, haemolysis of blood samples or delay in processing does not affect the measurement of urea.

Physiological aspects

Urea is produced exclusively by hepatic enzymes of the urea cycle and is the major nitrogen-containing metabolic product of protein catabolism in man. The kidney is responsible for excreting more than 90% of urea with losses through the skin and gastrointestinal tract accounting for the remainder. On an average protein diet urinary excretion of urea is 35–45 g (580–750 mmol)/day.

There is no evidence for active transport of urea by the kidney. It is freely filtered by the glomerulus but then is passively transported out of the proximal renal tubule into the interstitium under the influence of a concentration gradient established by water reabsorption. The small molecular weight, its ability to diffuse freely and its presence in generous amounts make urea a major factor among the contributors to the osmolar gradients generated in the kidney through the countercurrent mechanism. Under conditions of diuresis only 40% of the urea load is reabsorbed whereas in antidiuresis the amount reabsorbed increases to about 70%.

Urea measurements are used to help assess the adequacy of dialysis. Because it moves readily across the dialysis membrane it changes substantially through the course of the dialysis. A measurement pre- and post-dialysis (expressed as a reduction ratio) has become one of the accepted markers of adequacy of dialysis treatment.

Factors affecting the plasma urea without altering renal function

Reduced urine flow

A mild reduction in renal plasma flow results in reduced urine output without affecting the glomerular filtration rate. This same reduction may, however, significantly increase the plasma urea without changing the plasma creatinine concentration. Factors causing a reduced renal plasma flow include:

- mild dehydration. Fluid loss from any cause or excessive use of diuretics (particularly in the elderly when the signs may be subtle) is a common cause of mild dehydration. Serial body weights are a useful guide to changes in hydration. A high index of suspicion and a careful clinical history are necessary to come to a correct clinical assessment.
- cardiac failure. The reduction in cardiac output in congestive cardiac failure leads to a reduced renal plasma flow and urine flow rate. An improvement in cardiac function in this setting will be accompanied by a restoration of renal plasma flow and a return of the plasma urea concentration to baseline.

Altered urea production

Urea production is readily varied by altering the amount of protein available for metabolism and by drugs that affect the metabolic process. Examples of this are:

- gastrointestinal bleeding. Upper gastrointestinal bleeding will provide a protein 'meal' that may be substantial in size. The rise in plasma urea often precedes the passage of melena stools.
- dietary protein intake. Daily protein intake that in normal health may vary greatly on a day-to-day basis is a major factor in fluctuations seen in the plasma urea concentration. The plasma urea concentration may double in response to a change from a low to high protein intake and when renal function is abnormal this change may be three- or four-fold.
- metabolic state. Urea production is markedly increased in the presence of hypercatabolism such as is seen with infection, postoperatively or with trauma. An increased plasma urea concentration may be an early sign of unsuspected sepsis.
- drugs. Corticosteroids and tetracyclines (except doxycycline and minocycline) significantly increase protein catabolism and result in an increase in plasma urea concentration. These agents must be used with great caution in renal failure where further elevation of an already raised plasma urea concentration may lead to a vicious cycle of vomiting, dehydration and uraemia. Conversely androgens diminish urea production by inducing an anabolic state. These agents were used in the predialysis era to assist in the treatment of acute renal failure.
- liver disease. Urea production depends on the function of hepatic enzymes. In severe liver disease urea production may be affected but in practice this is seen only in the late stages of liver failure.

Obstruction

Partial obstruction of the urinary tract that results in a reduction of urine flow to less than 2 mL/min creates a situation similar to that seen with dehydration. Here the reduced urine flow rate allows more time for increased tubular reabsorption, leading to a reduced excretion of urea and a consequent rise in the plasma urea concentration without any change in the plasma creatinine concentration.

The ratio of plasma urea/plasma creatinine

The main advantage of plasma urea determinations lies in their comparison with plasma creatinine concentration. This is sometimes expressed as a plasma urea/creatinine ratio. While this means of expressing the results draws attention to some of the factors listed above, the ratio itself may be misleading, particularly when renal function is unstable or multiple clinical factors are evident. As a consequence the ratio does not have an established place in the clinical practice of most physicians.

Is the result abnormal?

The reference range for plasma urea in most laboratories is 2.5–6.4 mmol/L. The neonatal range is 0.5–1.0 mmol/L lower than in adults, and in adults over 60 years of age the normal range may be marginally higher than in younger adults. The concentration of plasma urea is slightly higher in males than in females.

What action is needed if the result is abnormal?

An abnormal plasma urea should always be pursued until an explanation for the abnormality is evident. The first step is to determine the renal function (by plasma creatinine measurement) and to compare the degree of elevation of urea and creatinine. If the elevation is comparable then one need look no further for an explanation and should follow the course outlined in the chapter *Plasma creatinine* in this book.

If the plasma urea is increased out of proportion to renal function, then the list of non-renal factors affecting the plasma urea (above) should be checked. These include symptoms of obstruction (e.g. voiding difficulties), dehydration (to be suspected if renal function is normal and the patient is on diuretics), cardiac failure, gastrointestinal bleeding and drugs. Dietary protein intake should be assessed and if found to exceed more than 2 g/kg/day should be suspected as the likely cause. If a likely cause is found, corrective action should be taken and the plasma urea checked again a few days later.

If a cause of an increased plasma urea (out of proportion to renal function) is not clinically evident, a 24-hour urine volume should be obtained. If the measured volume is below 1.5 L/day the effect of increasing fluid input to achieve a urine flow of more than 2.5 L/day should be determined. Obstruction should be excluded by ordering urinary tract imaging (initially ultrasound). Faeces should be tested for blood. While a hypercatabolic state is usually obvious, it may be present in the absence of fever, overt trauma or inflammation. Once the cause is suspected, corrective action should be taken with reassessment at a later date.

If the plasma urea is lower than normal, once again comparison with renal function should be made. The most common cause of a reduced plasma urea is a state of volume expansion such as occurs in pregnancy or in the presence of the syndrome of inappropriate secretion of antidiuretic hormone. Another common cause is a low protein intake, usually in the context of anorexia from any cause. Other possibilities to exclude are severe liver disease, polyuria (particularly that seen with compulsive water drinking) or an anabolic state associated with the use of androgenic steroids. These factors can usually be identified by the bedside.

Summary

The determination of plasma urea concentration will continue to be clinically important. If the plasma urea measurements are used with insight then they can contribute significantly to clinical management decisions. The plasma urea concentration or the urea clearance used on its own have no place in the determination of renal function. Used in conjunction with an assessment of renal function the plasma urea reflects the state of hydration and protein catabolic status, and is a guide to adequate protein nutrition.

Plasma sodium

16

T. H. Mathew

SYNOPSIS

Disorders of sodium metabolism are common in a hospital setting but are also seen in general practice. There is always an explanation to be found for important deviations of the sodium concentration from normal. The plasma sodium concentration itself cannot be used in isolation from the clinical setting. Determination of the fluid status of the patient is paramount in formulating a management plan. In all but the most severe disturbances of sodium metabolism, restoration of the plasma sodium concentration to the normal range should be accomplished slowly over a few days. Rapid correction, particularly of hyponatraemia, should be avoided as it may cause permanent cerebral damage.

Introduction

A plasma sodium concentration is one of the most frequently performed chemical tests. The measurement represents a ratio, determined equally by the amount of available sodium and water. The single most important fact to appreciate in assessing a plasma sodium result is that it cannot be used in isolation as an indicator of total body sodium excess or deficiency. The four basic disorders of water and sodium metabolism are:

1 hyponatraemia—a relative excess of water in relation to sodium
2 hypernatraemia—a relative deficit of water in relation to sodium
3 hypovolaemia—a reduction of extracellular fluid where total body sodium (salt) may be normal or reduced
4 oedema—a reflection of sodium excess and hypervolaemia.

In a hospital setting hyponatraemia is the commonest of these disorders but in general practice oedema is prevalent. Appropriate management is based on a thorough understanding of the relationship of sodium to water and the variables controlling these factors. Sodium is mainly found in the extracellular compartments of the body where its concentration is easily and quickly altered by changes in extracellular fluid volume (ECFV). The normal range of plasma sodium is 135–145 mmol/L.

Technical aspects

Plasma sodium is measured in the water phase of the plasma but is expressed in mmol/L of the whole plasma.
Pseudohyponatraemia is said to be present when the plasma sodium measurement is below normal but can be corrected in the laboratory to normal by the removal of excess protein or lipid from the plasma compartment of the sample. This condition is seen in paraproteinaemias or severe hyperlipidaemia where the plasma sodium concentration may be less than 120 mmol/L yet the true plasma water sodium concentration is 145 mmol/L. A plasma osmolality is a quick and easy way of checking for pseudohyponatraemia when it is suspected. The measurement of plasma osmolality is unaffected by protein and lipids which occupy space in the plasma sample. The sodium concentration may be reduced a small amount through this same mechanism by elevated levels of urea, mannitol or glucose and in this situation the osmolality of the plasma will be raised.

Physiological and clinical aspects

Once an abnormal plasma sodium result is to hand, the first step in management is to assess the ECFV. This can be satisfactorily accomplished at the bedside. An expanded ECFV should be suspected when there is dependent oedema, raised jugular venous pressure, pulmonary congestion and a third heart sound. A contracted ECFV (volume depletion) should be suspected when there is reduced tissue turgor, low jugular venous pressure, postural hypotension, and tachycardia and poor perfusion of peripheral tissues. Serial body weights are most helpful in confirming the clinical assessment of the state of volume load. Even with experience this assessment may be difficult, particularly in the elderly patient. It is common to observe up to 5% change in body weight from the baseline without any clinical evidence of fluid overload or depletion. The chest X-ray is a useful aid when the clinical signs leave uncertainty.

Hyponatraemia

Hyponatraemia is seldom of clinical significance when the plasma sodium is above 125 mmol/L despite the lower level of normal being set at 135 mmol/L. It is usually unnecessary to take urgent action till the level is less than 120 mmol/L. When the plasma sodium is 120–135 mmol/L, appropriate modification to oral water and sodium intake will lead to a gradual increase in the plasma sodium concentration.

An age over 70 years and a rapid rate of change of the sodium concentration increases the likelihood of symptoms from hyponatraemia. In a young healthy patient, a drop in plasma sodium to less than 125 mmol/L over a few hours may result in a depressed sensorium and the possibility of seizures whereas a plasma sodium of less than 110 mmol/L may be well tolerated, even in the elderly, when the decline occurs gradually over some weeks.

Symptoms attributable to hyponatraemia include lethargy, anorexia, cramps and confusion. Signs may include altered sensorium, depressed deep tendon reflexes, hypothermia and seizures.

Table 16.1 summarises the three main mechanisms, the effect on ECFV, and the causes and treatment of hyponatraemia. A notable cause, particularly in the elderly, is the combined use of thiazides with triamterene or amiloride. Severe hyponatraemia (down to less than 100 mmol/L) may develop as a new event even after many months of satisfactory therapy.

TABLE 16.1 Hyponatraemia

MECHANISM	ECFV	CAUSES	TREATMENT
Water retention	Mild increase (no oedema)	Excess water intake (intravenous fluids or compulsive water drinking)	Water restriction
Sodium and water deficiency with a larger deficit in sodium	Decreased	Urine loss –diuretics –Addison's –sodium losing –nephropathy GIT loss Skin loss –sweating –burns	Isotonic saline
Combined sodium and water excess with greater increase of water	Increased	(a) Circulating volume increased: –cardiac failure –renal failure (b) Circulating volume decreased: –nephrotic syndrome –cirrhosis	Diuretic (albumin infusion in severe hypo-albuminaemia)

Water retention

When hyponatraemia exists with a normal or mildly increased ECFV the diagnostic possibilities include drugs that stimulate antidiuretic hormone (ADH) or simulate its action. Examples of these are nicotine, carbamazepine, non-steroidal anti-inflammatory drugs and the Cox 2 inhibitors. Inappropriate secretion of ADH occurs in a number of conditions including carcinomas of the lung and the pancreas, pulmonary conditions (pneumonia, tuberculosis) and central nervous system disorders including stroke and infection.

Dehydration with sodium loss in excess of water

The combination of clinical dehydration and hyponatraemia is diagnostic of excessive loss of sodium from the gut, skin or urine. When the cause is not obvious then loss from the urinary tract (such as from undiagnosed polycystic disease or reflux nephropathy) should be the prime suspect. Adrenal insufficiency should be suspected if renal imaging is normal.

Fluid overload with water retention in excess of sodium

The hyponatremic patient with oedema must have cardiac or renal failure, cirrhosis or the nephrotic syndrome. With these latter two conditions the urine sodium will be low in the absence of exposure of the patient to diuretic therapy.

Hypernatraemia

Hypernatraemia is usually defined as a plasma sodium greater than 150 mmol/L. It is a less common condition than hyponatraemia. Renal concentrating defects do not of themselves usually result in hypernatraemia. It is necessary to add to these conditions a disturbance in the thirst mechanism or to limit access to oral fluids. Hypernatraemia tends to be seen only in the young, the elderly and the sick. The thirst mechanism is very effective in preventing hypernatraemia with oral intake frequently rising to about 10 L/24 hours in conditions such as diabetes insipidus.

Table 16.2 summarises the mechanisms, effect on ECFV, and the causes and treatment of hypernatraemia.

The clinical signs and symptoms of hypernatraemia are mainly neurological and are due to shrinkage of the brain cells. In severe cases structural damage (tearing of vessels, venous sinus thrombosis) has been reported. An acute rise in plasma sodium concentration is of more concern than a slow and steady rise, with a considerable mortality being experienced when the sodium exceeds 160 mmol/L.

The earliest signs of hypernatraemia are restlessness, irritability and lethargy and the signs are tremor, twitching and ataxia. The elderly and the very young are more susceptible to a given level of hypernatraemia and the clinical changes are more severe when the rise occurs over a few hours or days.

TABLE 16.2 Hypernatraemia

MECHANISM	ECFV	CAUSES	TREATMENT
Sodium and water loss with water loss predominant	Decreased	Renal loss: osmotic diuresis Extrarenal loss: −excessive sweating −diarrhoea	Hypotonic saline
Pure water loss	Normal or minimal decrease	Renal loss: diabetes insipidus −nephrogenic −central Extrarenal loss: respiratory and skin	Water replenishment
Sodium intake excessive	Increased	Hypertonic input (intravenous, dialysis, oral) Primary aldosteronism Cushing's syndrome	Diuretics and water replenishment

A reading of more than 160 mmol/L is a medical emergency when accompanied by only minor symptoms and signs because the situation can deteriorate rapidly with the onset of seizures leading to death. A plasma sodium concentration of less than 150 mmol/L is seldom of concern though an attempt should be made to diagnose the cause and to take corrective action.

Combined loss of sodium and water with water loss predominant

Body fluid loss that is hypotonic (sweating, polyuria) is usually associated with an intact thirst mechanism and therefore the tendency to hypernatraemia will be corrected by extra water intake. It is only when there is restricted access to water (such as when a person is elderly and bedridden) or if the thirst mechanism is impaired that hypernatraemia will occur.

An osmotic diuresis as a cause of hypernatraemia may be driven by glucose (particularly in uncontrolled diabetes with a drowsy non-ketotic hyperosmolar patient), urea in recovering acute renal failure or by mannitol such as in a forced diuresis protocol. The tube-feeding syndrome has disappeared as a cause of hypernatraemia due to the recognition that adequate water is essential in any enteral high protein-feeding regimen.

Water loss with no sodium loss
This condition is seen only when renal concentrating defects that affect water reabsorption are present. The cause may be 'central' diabetes insipidus where the production of ADH from the posterior pituitary is deficient, or 'renal' as in nephrogenic diabetes insipidus. In this condition, the response of the renal tubule to normal amounts of ADH is impaired. The causes of nephrogenic diabetes insipidus are numerous and include renal disease (analgesic nephropathy, medullary cystic disease), drugs (lithium, amphotericin, colchicines), electrolyte deficiency (hypokalaemia, hypocalcaemia), or other causes (myeloma, amyloidosis).

The clinical signs will be mainly of hypernatraemia rather than fluid loss for two-thirds of the water loss is borne by the intracellular compartment, as the membrane is freely permeable to water. Thus the ECFV shows only minor signs of dehydration.

Excessive sodium intake
This infrequent cause of hypernatraemia results from the excessive administration of sodium-containing fluids (by any route) and manifests clinically as both fluid overload and hypernatraemia. Primary aldosteronism and, to a lesser extent, Cushing's syndrome cause a similar situation but are characterised by an 'escape' mechanism leading to only minor degrees of fluid overload and mild hypernatraemia.

Is the result abnormal?

The normal limits of plasma sodium are clearly defined at 135–145 mmol/L. The difficulty, as discussed throughout this chapter, is to decide which values outside these limits are clinically meaningful. The important aspects in deciding the meaning of an individual result and in determining a course of action are the clinical state of the patient, the rate of change of the plasma sodium concentration and, finally, the absolute reading. There is no fixed clinical response to a reading of, say, 122 mmol/L. In one patient simple correction to water intake is appropriate and in another urgent intravenous saline and other initiatives are indicated.

What action is needed if the result is abnormal?
Hyponatraemia

The first step is to assess the state of the ECFV by clinical means. Table 16.1 summarises the diagnostic possibilities. Treatment depends on the cause and the clinical situation. In states of water retention, restriction of oral water intake will suffice. In overload states diuretics combined with water restriction will correct both the fluid overload and the hyponatraemia. In volume depletion, therapy will consist of replenishment with sodium and water. This may often be accomplished orally but when the loss is from the gastrointestinal route, intravenous therapy is usually required. Replenishment should be with isotonic saline that will allow gradual correction of the hyponatraemia.

Rapid correction of hyponatraemia should be avoided unless the clinical situation is compelling. There is very little place for hypertonic saline (e.g. 3% saline) that may lead not only to fluid overload but also to cerebral disturbance that may be permanent. An appropriate program is one that leads to correction of the plasma sodium concentration to the normal range within the next 2–3 days.

Hypernatraemia

Again, the first step is to assess the state of the ECFV by the bedside and to consider the clinical possibilities. Simple observations such as the daily urine volume and measurement of the urinary sodium will clarify the diagnosis. Therapy depends on the cause of hypernatraemia. When the diagnosis is predominant water loss, removal of the offending drug, correction of the electrolyte abnormality and administration of ADH may be helpful. Water replenishment will, in addition, hasten the return of the plasma sodium concentration to less than 150 mmol/L. When sodium administration has been excessive, diuretics combined with liberal water administration will be helpful. When the cause has been water loss combined with sodium loss, hypotonic saline is indicated.

The plan should be to return the plasma sodium concentration to near the normal range within a few days. An acceptable rule of thumb is to achieve 50% of the necessary correction in 24 hours, with the remaining 50% being accomplished over the next 2 days.

Summary

The management of plasma sodium abnormalities is basically logical and straightforward and is based on an understanding of normal sodium handling. The clinical possibilities to explain the various combinations of fluid state and sodium status are not great in number. The overriding consideration in appropriate management is to formulate a plan aimed at correcting the sodium and fluid status over some days rather than hours. The approach outlined above is applicable and will solve the vast majority of sodium abnormalities presenting to the practitioner in or out of hospital.

17 | The red cells

W. R. Pitney
Updated by R. A. Dunstan

Introduction

A complete (or full) blood count (CBC) is one of the most commonly requested of all laboratory tests. It forms part of all multiphasic screening procedures and it is requested almost routinely in any patient with more than a minor illness. A CBC is performed using an automated laboratory instrument which measures the number of red cells, leucocytes and platelets and generates a number of indices and often an automated leucocyte differential count.

Technical aspects

Three measurements in the report refer to the red cells—the haemoglobin concentration, the red cell count and the haematocrit (or packed cell volume). From these three, the red cell indices can be calculated: the mean cell volume (MCV), mean cell haemoglobin (MCH), mean cell haemoglobin concentration (MCHC) (Table 17.1) and red cell distribution width (RDW). The RDW is a mathematical representation of the variability in size of the erythrocyte population. The erythrocytes are categorised by volume as they are counted in automated cell counting equipment. Most modern instruments measure the MCV and calculate the PCV. The laboratory report should also provide a comment on the morphological appearance of the red cells in the stained blood film.

The most important aspects of the blood count report are the haemoglobin value and the comment on the blood film, and these should always be considered together.

TABLE 17.1 Measurements and red cell indices			
MEASUREMENTS	**INDICES**	**CALCULATION OF INDICES**	
Haemoglobin concentration (Hb, g/L)	Mean cell volume (MCV)	$\dfrac{\text{PCV}}{\text{RCC}}$	expressed as femtolitres (fL, 10^{-15} L)
Red cell count (RCC, X 10^{12}/L)	Mean cell haemoglobin (MCH)	$\dfrac{\text{Hb}}{\text{RCC}}$	expressed as picograms (pg, 10^{-12} g)
Haematocrit or packed cell volume (PCV, L/L)	Mean cell haemoglobin concentration (MCHC)	$\dfrac{\text{Hb}}{\text{PCV}}$	expressed as g/L

Is the result abnormal?

The abnormality reported may be an increase or a decrease in haemoglobin value, red cell count or haematocrit outside the normal ranges, and there may be morphological changes in the red cells in the blood film. There may also be abnormalities in the red cell indices but these should correlate with the red cell morphology, e.g. hypochromia should be associated with a low MCHC. Minor degrees of anisocytosis (variation in size) and poikilocytosis (variation in shape) are not significant, and are found in normal people. A low haemoglobin value due to leukaemia or other malignant blood disorders will usually be associated with abnormalities in white cells and platelets, and the blood film comment should indicate the diagnosis. It will be assumed in what follows that any abnormalities in the blood film are confined to the red cells.

Low haemoglobin, red cells normal

The patient appears to have a normocytic, normochromic anaemia and the red cell indices are in the normal range. It is important to remember that the normal range of haemoglobin concentration is less in children and in pregnancy. Women of child-bearing age usually have haemoglobin values about 20 g/L lower than men, but this difference becomes less after the menopause. Normochromic, normocytic anaemia is often a reflection of a general medical or surgical disorder. The patient should be assessed with regard to the conditions listed in Table 17.2. The blood sedimentation rate is commonly elevated in these conditions and it provides useful information on disease activity. Following haemorrhage and in some types of haemolytic anaemia, the red cells may be of normal size and shape, but the film report may comment on polychromasia, which indicates increased release of reticulocytes from the bone marrow, and a reticulocyte count should be performed. Haemolytic anaemia is often associated with blood film comments such as the presence of spherocytosis and autoagglutination. A comment of increased red cell rouleaux suggests the possibility of multiple myeloma. A bone marrow examination is usually necessary if there is no obvious cause for normochromic, normocytic anaemia.

TABLE 17.2 Important causes of normochromic, normocytic anaemia

Renal failure
Hypothyroidism
Aplasia
Chronic infection
Acute blood loss
Haemolysis
Rheumatoid arthritis
Occult malignancy
Multiple myeloma

Low haemoglobin, red cells hypochromic

Usually all three calculated red cell indices will be reduced. The most common cause is iron deficiency anaemia, but the alternative diagnosis of thalassaemia trait should be considered, especially in patients of Mediterranean extraction. In such patients, further investigation is always warranted, since hypochromia may indicate either iron deficiency or thalassaemia trait. The MCV is usually lower and the red cell count higher in thalassaemia trait than in iron deficiency, and stipple cells and target cells may be prominent features of the blood film report. Haemoglobin studies and serum iron determination will establish the correct diagnosis. Clinical judgement *is* required to determine whether a patient with iron deficiency warrants further investigation. Menorrhagia and repeated pregnancies are common causes in women of child-bearing age. A site of occult blood loss must always be suspected when iron deficiency is diagnosed in men or in postmenopausal women. Carcinoma of the caecum presents classically as iron deficiency anaemia. A rare cause of hypochromic anaemia in the elderly is sideroblastic anaemia; bone marrow examination is necessary for diagnosis.

Low haemoglobin, red cells macrocytic

The MCV and MCH will be elevated, but the MCHC should be normal. Macrocytosis occurs in liver disease (when the macrocytic cells are usually round and may show a target-cell appearance) and in megaloblastic anaemia (when there is usually prominent poikilocytosis, and ovalling of cells). The usual causes of megaloblastic anaemia are nutritional (folate deficiency) or pernicious anaemia (vitamin B_{12} deficiency). Bone marrow examination and measurement of serum B_{12} and folate are indicated. Figure 17.1 summarises the investigation of the anaemias.

Raised haemoglobin

An elevated haemoglobin value may be a temporary phenomenon due to haemoconcentration, e.g. dehydration from excessive use of diuretics. Patients with chronic bronchitis and cigarette smokers may have a moderate elevation of haemoglobin. In cigarette smokers, this is due to the inhalation of carbon monoxide and the formation of carboxyhaemoglobin which shifts the oxygen dissociation curve of haemoglobin to the left. Cessation of smoking may result in a considerable fall in haemoglobin value over a period of 6–8 weeks. A reduced plasma volume with a normal red cell mass (stress polycythaemia or spurious

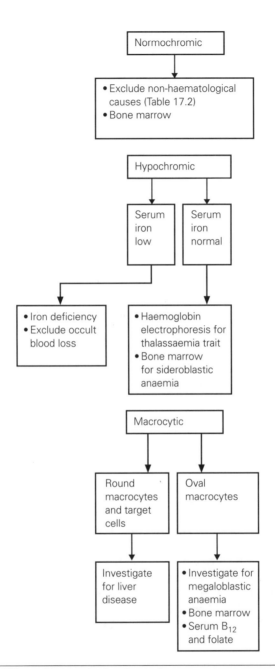

FIGURE 17. 1 The investigation of anaemia

polycythaemia) sometimes occurs in middle-aged males for no apparent reason. True polycythaemia may be primary or secondary. If the white cells and platelets are normal and there is no splenomegaly, the patient should be investigated for causes of secondary polycythaemia. A blood volume determination is usually necessary to distinguish between secondary polycythaemia and spurious polycythaemia.

Summary

An abnormality in the blood count always warrants careful consideration. It is unlikely to be due to laboratory error, as most laboratories now use automated blood cell counters with a high degree of accuracy and with good methods of quality control. It should be remembered, however, that the quoted normal ranges for haemoglobin, red cell count and haematocrit are too rigid to include all normal people, and an occasional result outside the normal range may not be abnormal. Furthermore, the normal ranges quoted by different laboratories show some variation. *Anaemia is a laboratory finding, not a disease entity, and it is imperative that the cause be found before treatment is commenced. The use of haematinics or blood transfusion without proper characterisation of anaemia is not good practice and it makes subsequent investigation more difficult.*

FURTHER READING

Beal R. W. Anaemia: the cause dictates treatment. *Curr Ther* 1978; 19: 69–74.

Matthews J. R. D. Haematological tests. *Patient Manage* 1979; 3 (Jun): 45–59.

18 | Interpretation of biochemical tests for iron deficiency: diagnostic difficulties related to limitations of individual tests

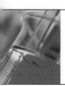

F. Firkin and B. Rush

SYNOPSIS

Biochemical tests for iron deficiency have a particular place for evaluating the cause of microcytic anaemia (a mean red cell corpuscular volume less than 80 fL), and are also important for assessment of the contribution of iron deficiency to anaemia in which there are multiple contributory factors. Microcytic anaemia is most commonly due to iron deficiency, but is also caused by thalassaemia, and can occur in some patients with anaemia secondary to chronic infection, inflammation, or malignancy (anaemia of chronic disease), even though the majority of these patients have a normal mean corpuscular volume (MCV). It is essential to recognise that results of tests of iron status are relatively frequently distorted by other clinical factors. This can occur to an extent which provides a misleading view of iron reserves unless the impact of these factors is recognised by utilising the combined results of currently available tests to obtain a more reliable overview of the situation than is provided by any individual test. Currently available tests are, however, effective in providing a reliable index of iron status sufficiently frequently that it is not appropriate to perform endoscopic examinations merely because a patient has anaemia, especially normocytic anaemia, unless there are biochemical indices of iron deficiency, or highly suggestive clinical indications of gastrointestinal disease.

Investigation of iron status

The bracket of tests covered under Item 66263 in the Australian Medicare Benefits Schedule of (a) serum iron, (b) transferrin or iron-binding capacity and (c) ferritin, represent an appropriate first-line approach for investigation of iron deficiency.

Pathophysiological aspects
Serum or plasma iron/transferrin relationships

The serum (or plasma) iron level falls progressively below the normal range (about 14–32 µmol per litre) when the amount of iron in the body decreases further after the reserves of iron have become exhausted. The level in the serum or plasma of transferrin, the major iron-transporting protein in the circulation, rises under these circumstances towards, or above, the upper limit of the normal range. A subnormal level of iron in association with a supranormal level of transferrin is very strong evidence of iron deficiency.

Levels of iron and transferrin in the serum, however, fall rapidly as part of the acute phase response after onset of the inflammatory process despite the presence of normal iron stores. This abnormality persists as long as the inflammatory process is sustained, and is classically associated with the development of anaemia of chronic disease. A low serum iron level in this setting is unfortunately frequently misinterpreted as evidence of iron deficiency, a major diagnostic error that can be avoided by simultaneous examination of the transferrin level, which in this context is subnormal, or in the low normal range. Estimation of the level of serum iron alone is consequently inadvisable. The loss of diagnostic specificity of a low level of serum iron for iron deficiency in the presence of inflammatory processes and certain other forms of chronic disease is usually revealed by an inappropriately low level of concurrently estimated transferrin. (See Table 18.1 on page 112.)

Relation of transferrin level to total iron-binding capacity of serum

Transferrin is the carrier protein which binds most of the iron present in serum, and its concentration is estimated by

TABLE 18.1 Problems in interpretation of serum iron levels in relation to body iron stores

FALSE NORMAL	FALSE LOW
Recent iron medication, possibly unappreciated as a component in vitamins with mineral supplements	Concurrent acute or chronic inflammation Postoperative Concurrent infection Malignancy Hypoproteinaemia

immunological assays which demonstrate the level in the serum of adults is about 1.9 to 3.1 g per litre. The functional capacity of transferrin is represented by the total amount of iron that can be bound to serum protein, so that total iron-binding capacity provides an alternative view of the concentration of transferrin in serum. (See Table 18.2.)

TABLE 18.2 Problems in interpretation of serum transferrin levels in relation to body iron stores

FALSE LOW	FALSE NORMAL
Concurrent acute and chronic disease	Hypoproteinaemia

Expression of results as percentage saturation of transferrin

The extent to which the iron-binding sites on transferrin are occupied by iron is calculated by dividing the serum iron level by either the directly measured level of serum total iron-binding capacity, or by the value for serum iron-binding capacity extrapolated from the transferrin level. The percentage saturation of these sites is normally 20–50%. The view has been expressed that a subnormal percentage saturation is a useful index of iron deficiency, but low values are also obtained in chronic disorders, and the expression consequently lacks specificity.

Assessment of serum ferritin

The level of ferritin in serum bears a direct relationship to the amount of iron in the iron stores of the body, and subnormal values can be detected when body iron stores are exhausted even before the serum iron level has substantially declined. The 'normal' range is methodology-, age- and sex-related with values, for example, of 25–155 µg/L quoted for menstruating adult females. Values are greater in males and are lower in children. There is a high degree of specificity in the relation of a subnormal ferritin level and iron deficiency, but in iron-deficient subjects some clinical states can increase the level of ferritin in the circulation to the normal range. (See Table 18.3.)

TABLE 18.3 Problems in interpretation of serum ferritin levels in relation to body iron stores

FALSE LOW	FALSE NORMAL
Very uncommon	Concurrent acute and chronic disorders
	Hepatocellular damage
	Some malignancies

Examples of interpretation of test results

Example A

A 23-year-old man with longstanding microcytic anaemia unresponsive to oral iron supplements.

Hb 89 g/L, MCV 57 fL (N 80–96)
Serum iron < 3 micromol/L (N 14–32)
Serum transferrin 1.5 g/L (N 2.0–3.6)
Serum ferritin 195 µg/L (N 40–260)

The pattern of the iron study results is consistent with the effects of chronic inflammation. Subsequent determination of the erythrocyte sedimentation rate revealed a very high value of 119 mm/hour. An inflammatory disease was diagnosed and, after the underlying disorder responded to specific treatment, the haemoglobin level rose to 160 g/L and the MCV to normal.

Example B

A 47-year-old mother of a child with beta thalassaemia minor was found on testing of the family for evidence of thalassaemia to be anaemic.

Hb 65 g/L, MCV 59 fL (N 80–96)
Serum iron 5.3 micromol/L (N 14–32)
Serum transferrin 4.6 g/L (N 2.0–3.6)
Serum ferritin < 5 µg/L (N 25–155)

The pattern of the iron study results is typical of severe iron deficiency. The haemoglobin level and MCV returned to normal after iron replacement therapy and subsequent studies revealed no evidence of thalassaemia minor.

Summary
Value of combined test results in complex situations

Coexisting disease can make it impossible to assess iron status with biochemical tests in some instances, but concurrent determination of all three indices make it unlikely for an incorrect diagnosis of iron deficiency to be made, and in most instances provides a reliable index of body iron stores.

Further evaluation in inconclusive situations

In the absence of unequivocal data on the status of iron reserves where such information is of major clinical importance, it is possible to assess iron reserves by performing a bone marrow aspirate. The marrow particles are stained for iron with the Prussian Blue reaction. A negative result is considered to be the gold standard for iron deficiency, but the procedure is uncomfortable and is thus rarely performed.

An alternative approach is assessment of response to oral iron administration. A rise in the MCV, and an increase of more than 10 g/L in the haemoglobin level within 4 to 6 weeks is evidence that deficiency of iron is contributing to the anaemia. Trials of iron supplements are, however, usually unrewarding in normocytic anaemia where an alternative mechanism is usually responsible for the anaemia.

Appropriate use of tests for folate and vitamin B$_{12}$ deficiency

J. Metz

SYNOPSIS

A full blood count which shows anaemia and macrocytosis should prompt the practitioner to look for a deficiency of vitamin B$_{12}$ or folate. Tests commonly used for the detection of these vitamin deficiencies are serum folate, red cell folate and serum B$_{12}$ concentrations. Serum folate becomes subnormal in the early stages of negative folate balance, before reduction of folate stores. Red cell folate is a direct measure of tissue folate stores. Measurement of both serum and red cell folate yields the maximum information, but in practice, red cell folate needs to be assayed only when there is macrocytosis and the serum folate is low. Serum B$_{12}$ is a sensitive index of deficiency, but a low level does not necessarily indicate deficiency. Following the identification of folate or B$_{12}$ deficiency, a cause must be sought.

Introduction

Laboratory tests for folate and vitamin B$_{12}$ are essential for the diagnosis of a deficiency of these vitamins, and for the investigation of some forms of anaemia. Untreated, deficiency of folate or B$_{12}$ may lead to severe anaemia and, in B$_{12}$ deficiency, crippling neurological disease. The clinical indications for testing are broad (Table 19.1). Often the indication for testing is an abnormality found in a full blood examination, such as unexplained anaemia or macrocytosis. Neurological conditions associated with B_{12} deficiency include peripheral neuropathy and subacute combined degeneration of the spinal cord. Deterioration in cognitive ability may also occur. Serum B_{12} should therefore be checked, even in the absence of haematological abnormality, in patients with some unexplained neurological or neuropsychiatric abnormalities.

TABLE 19.1 Indications for which testing for folate and B_{12} deficiency might be considered

Unexplained anaemia
Macrocytosis
Suspected malabsorption
Some neurological diseases e.g. peripheral neuropathy
Some psychiatric disorders e.g. unexplained memory loss or dementia
Malnutrition, including subjects on restrictive diets, e.g. vegetarians
Haematological disease associated with increased cell turnover
Alcohol abuse
Drug therapy, e.g. anticonvulsants
Family history of pernicious anaemia
Infertility

Investigation of folate and vitamin B_{12} status

Three tests are in common use:
1 serum folate
2 red cell folate
3 serum vitamin B_{12}.

In addition, investigations should always include a full blood examination with assessment of a blood film.

The blood tests must always be taken before specific therapy begins. After such therapy, it may be impossible to identify the underlying deficiency.

Serum and red cell folate

The usual first test for folate deficiency is assay of serum folate (reference range 7–40 nmol/L). (Reference ranges for serum folate, red cell folate and serum vitamin B_{12} are specific to the methodology used by individual laboratories and may not be identical to the ranges given in the text.) The margin of safety between folate intake and requirement is small so the serum folate concentration may become subnormal after only 3 weeks of negative balance (folate intake less than folate consumption). This is a stage which precedes, and may not necessarily ever progress to, body folate depletion with subsequent haematological changes. Subnormal serum folate concentration may imply body deficiency, but the serum folate level depends on recent dietary intake and is not strictly a diagnostic test for body folate depletion. For example, a low serum folate concentration without body depletion occurs with recent alcohol abuse (Table 19.2).

TABLE 19.2 Problems in interpretation of serum and red cell folate levels in relation to body folate stores

	FALSE NORMAL	FALSE LOW
SERUM FOLATE	Patient given folic acid	Negative dietary folate balance Recent alcohol intake
RED CELL FOLATE	Following blood transfusion	Primary B_{12} deficiency

Red cell folate (reference range 360–1400 nmol/L) is a direct measure of tissue folate stores. It falls after about 4 months of negative folate balance. Red cell folate will differentiate between negative folate balance and body folate depletion. Low serum with normal red cell folate suggests negative folate balance. Subnormal values for both tests indicate tissue depletion.

A low concentration of red cell folate usually implies significant depletion of folate stores. Subnormal values may also occur in severe vitamin B_{12} deficiency, and return to normal following vitamin B_{12} therapy alone. A falsely normal result may occur in a folate-deficient patient who has received a blood transfusion (Table 19.2).

Measurement of serum folate only will not differentiate between negative folate balance and tissue folate depletion. Measurement of red cell folate *only* may miss the early stage of negative folate balance. Serum and red cell folate yield complementary data and together the maximum information. However, in practice, it is usual to 'screen' with the serum folate assay and to proceed to red cell folate only if the serum folate is subnormal. In a folate-deficient patient recently given folic acid, only red cell folate will detect deficiency.

Serum folate assay is technically easy to perform, and is reasonably reproducible, but falsely elevated values may occur in folate-deficient patients who have been given folic acid. For technical reasons, measurement of red cell folate is not as reliable or reproducible as serum folate.

Serum vitamin B_{12}

The most widely used test for B_{12} deficiency is the serum B_{12} assay (reference range 150–600 pmol/L). This is a sensitive index for the detection of B_{12} deficiency, but a low concentration does not necessarily indicate tissue deficiency. Conditions where the serum concentrations are low without tissue deficiency include pregnancy, folate deficiency, iron deficiency, simple atrophic gastritis, vegetarian diet, women taking oral contraceptives, and certain rare inherited disorders of B_{12} metabolism (Table 19.3). Concentrations below 150 pmol/L are sometimes seen in people (often elderly) who have no neurological or haematological abnormalities, eat a mixed diet and absorb B_{12} normally. Long-term observation indicates that the majority of these people do not develop clinical or haematological features of B_{12} deficiency. The cause of their low B_{12} is unknown, but low values should never be regarded as normal for the elderly.

The clinical significance of serum B_{12} levels that are only mildly reduced or in the region of 150–200 pmol/L may be difficult to determine. The presence of any haematological or neuropsychiatric evidence of B_{12} deficiency would indicate true B_{12} depletion and the need for B_{12} therapy. Although the serum B_{12} assay is generally reliable and reproducible, a result which does not appear compatible with the clinical findings should always be confirmed by repeat testing. A low serum B_{12} result should never be ignored.

Blood count and film examination

Changes in the blood count and film are relatively late manifestations of folate or B_{12} deficiency, but are often the first clues

TABLE 19.3 Problems in interpretation of serum B$_{12}$ levels in relation to body B$_{12}$ stores

FALSE NORMAL	FALSE LOW
Patient given B$_{12}$	Pregnancy
Myeloproliferative disease	Primary folate deficiency
Hepatoma	Iron deficiency
Acute liver disease	Inherited disorders of B$_{12}$
Inherited disorders of B$_{12}$	metabolism
metabolism	Some normal subjects
	?Oral contraceptives

to the deficiency. Folate and B$_{12}$ deficiency cannot be differentiated, as the haematological changes are identical. The degree of anaemia varies, but macrocytosis (raised mean cell volume—MCV) and hypersegmented neutrophils are important features. Many laboratories do not regard macrocytosis as significant until the MCV is greater than 100 fL, but in normal people the MCV should not be more than 95 fL, and a mild increase above this size may be the earliest haematological sign of deficiency. If there is associated iron deficiency or thalassaemia, the MCV will often not be raised, despite severe folate or B$_{12}$ deficiency. In addition, while macrocytosis is an important feature of folate or B$_{12}$ deficiency, it occurs in many other conditions such as alcohol abuse, liver disease, hypothyroidism and with some drugs, including oral contraceptives. Macrocytosis may be physiological in pregnancy and the newborn.

Bone marrow biopsy

In the past, bone marrow was commonly examined to confirm megaloblastic anaemia when folate or B$_{12}$ deficiency was suspected. Nowadays, with the ready availability of vitamin assays, this expensive and invasive procedure is less frequently used. It is of most value in differentiating macrocytosis due to myelodysplasia (preleukaemia) and erythroleukaemia from megaloblastic anaemia.

Identifying the deficient vitamin in macrocytic anaemia

In the investigation of patients with macrocytic anaemia, it is essential to assay both serum B$_{12}$ and serum and red cell folate in view of the reciprocal changes which may take place in the tests (Table 19.2). As red cell folate may fall moderately in patients with B_{12} deficiency, this test alone will not differentiate folate from B_{12} deficiency. Serum folate levels may be elevated, normal, or occasionally reduced in B_{12} deficiency. Furthermore, serum B_{12} levels may be reduced moderately in patients with folate deficiency. These parallel changes make it difficult to distinguish the combined deficiency of the two vitamins that may occur in malnutrition or with intestinal disorders.

Metabolic assays

The activities of folate and B_{12} in metabolic pathways generate various metabolites. Assay of these metabolites has been used in the diagnosis of folate and B_{12} deficiency. Serum homocysteine (Hcy) is raised in both folate and B_{12} deficiency. Although a sensitive index, it has limited specificity because elevations occur in other inherited and acquired disorders, particularly renal impairment. In view of the interest in elevated Hcy concentrations as a risk factor for cardiovascular disease, some laboratories now offer Hcy assays routinely. This assay may help when vitamin measurements are in the indeterminate range or do not correlate with the clinical findings. A normal Hcy level excludes significant folate or B_{12} deficiency.

Establishing the cause of the deficiency

After folate or B_{12} deficiency has been identified by suitable tests, a cause for the deficiency must be sought. Folate deficiency is commonly the result of undernutrition or malnutrition in association with increased demand (e.g. pregnancy). It is important to assess dietary folate intake and to exclude gluten enteropathy (coeliac disease). Dietary fads or reliance on 'junk' foods devoid of green vegetables, an important source of folate[1], renders members of all socioeconomic groups susceptible to deficiency.

Pernicious anaemia is the most important syndrome of B_{12} deficiency. The diagnosis identifies the need for lifelong B_{12} treatment and the maintenance of a high index of suspicion for complications such as carcinoma of the stomach. In the past, the diagnosis was usually established by assessing B_{12} absorption with the Schilling test, but this is not often used nowadays. However, valuable information can be obtained from blood tests for intrinsic factor antibodies (IFA), parietal cell antibodies (PCA) and serum gastrin assay. The presence of IFA is virtually diagnostic of pernicious anaemia, but they are detected in only about 50% of cases. PCA and elevated serum gastrin are common, but they are not diagnostic. In patients in whom IFA and PCA are not detected and serum gastrin is not elevated, the cause of the B_{12} deficiency is unlikely to be pernicious anaemia. It is controversial as to whether further investigation is warranted before treating these patients. The Schilling test is useful in this group to distinguish intrinsic factor deficiency from intestinal malabsorption.

REFERENCE

1   Stanton R. Dietary sources of essential vitamins. *Aust Prescr* 1992;
    15: 80–5.

20 | Tests of haemostasis: detection of the patient at risk of bleeding

J. McPherson and A. Street

SYNOPSIS

Acquired bleeding disorders are common. They complicate well-defined clinical disorders which can be detected by history and examination. Inherited bleeding disorders are uncommon, but can be detected by careful clinical assessment, including family history. Clinical assessment has high sensitivity, although low specificity, for the presence of a bleeding disorder. In contrast, both the sensitivity and specificity of routine laboratory screening are low. Both false negative and false positive results are common with the basic laboratory 'screening tests'. In a patient without a suggestive history, these tests are inappropriate. In a patient with a suggestive history, they may well be inadequate.

Introduction

Normal haemostasis involves two processes:

1 platelet adhesion to areas of vascular injury with the subsequent formation of a platelet thrombus
2 surface or tissue-contact mediated activation of coagulation with sequential enzymic reactions culminating in the formation of a fibrin thrombus.

These two processes are interactive, although their dominance varies in different sites of the vascular system. Activation of haemostasis is accompanied by activation of the fibrinolytic system which should eventually achieve partial or complete removal of the thrombus.

Clinically important abnormalities of these mechanisms are common and a logical and cost-effective approach to the detection of patients at risk of bleeding is required.

Clinical assessment
Acquired bleeding disorders

These disorders occur in well-defined clinical settings and the history and physical examination are sensitive screens for these problems. The commonest cause of an acquired bleeding disorder is drug therapy:

- *aspirin or other non-steroidal anti-inflammatory drug (NSAID)* causing platelet dysfunction. The occurrence and severity of bleeding is variable.
- *cytotoxic drugs* causing thrombocytopenia
- *oral anticoagulant therapy* inhibiting the synthesis of the vitamin K-dependent coagulation factors.

Various disorders may also be associated with a bleeding tendency:

- *Chronic liver disease* can result in a variety of haemostatic abnormalities ranging from deficiency of vitamin K-dependent coagulation factors, through more global coagulation factor deficiencies to low-grade disseminated intravascular coagulation (DIC).
- Patients with *renal failure* may have significant platelet dysfunction.
- Those with *myeloproliferative disorders* may also have significant abnormalities of platelet function.
- Patients with *lymphoproliferative or autoimmune disease* may develop autoantibodies to coagulation factors or platelets.
- Paraproteins in patients with *plasma cell dyscrasias* may interfere with platelet function or fibrin formation.

Inherited bleeding disorders

These disorders are less common and the vast majority of patients will have a personal and/or family history of excessive bleeding.

The history is a sensitive, though not specific, screen for these patients. It is important to enquire into bleeding during and after surgical or dental procedures; a return to the operating theatre, blood transfusion, or a need for packing or suture of dental sockets would increase the likelihood of an underlying problem.

Menorrhagia, recurrent epistaxis and easy bruising are sensitive indicators, although associated with a high rate of false positives. The perception of menstrual blood loss is variable and often influenced by family norms; the frequency of pad/tampon change may assist in determining its significance. Menorrhagia commencing after pregnancies and childbirth and uninfluenced by hormone supplements is unlikely to be due to an inherited haemostatic disorder. Peripartum bleeding is rare in patients with von Willebrand's disease (arguably the most common inherited haemostatic disorder) and the absence of such a history should not influence the decision as to whether investigation is required.

'Spontaneous' haemarthroses and major muscle bleeds are characteristic of haemophilia A (factor VIII deficiency) or B (factor IX deficiency).

Gastrointestinal bleeding and/or epistaxis as isolated problems are unlikely to be due to an inherited bleeding disorder. However, mucosal surfaces should always be inspected for the characteristic lesions of hereditary haemorrhagic telangiectasia. This condition is underdiagnosed.

If a positive family history is obtained, the pattern of affected individuals may suggest autosomal (e.g. von Willebrand's disease) or X-linked (e.g. haemophilia) inheritance.

Bleeding time (BT)

The skin bleeding time reflects 'primary haemostasis', the interaction of platelets with arterioles and capillaries to form a platelet plug. The test is rarely useful and should not be performed if the platelet count is less than 100×10^9/L and if the patient has taken aspirin in the preceding 7–10 days, or a NSAID in the past 1–4 days (depending on the half-life of the specific drug). Although the effect of these drugs on the bleeding time is variable, their use renders a prolonged bleeding time uninterpretable. If the result will be uninterpretable, the test should not be done. As patients may not be aware of the aspirin content of prescribed or over-the-counter medications, both the requesting doctor and the laboratory should check the drug history before testing.

The bleeding time may be abnormal in acquired and inherited disorders of platelet function, von Willebrand's disease, the rare afibrinogenaemias and inherited disorders of collagen. It may also be prolonged in patients with 'senile purpura', but the test is neither appropriate nor useful in this condition.

The value of the bleeding time as a 'screening test' of haemostasis is severely limited by its lack of specificity and sensitivity and its use cannot be recommended. The lack of specificity is the result of its susceptibility to physiological and technical variables. This so-called 'standardised' technique varies between laboratories and between operators within a given laboratory. It is also an insensitive test and may be normal in patients with mild to moderate von Willebrand's disease and in those with disorders of platelet function. Although the BT can be prolonged by aspirin and other NSAIDs, is often abnormal in uraemia and may be abnormal in patients with myeloproliferative disorders, the presence and degree of an abnormality do not correlate with the risk of bleeding. The test cannot be recommended as a predictor of surgical bleeding.[1]

Activated partial thromboplastin time (APTT)

The APTT reflects the activity of coagulation factors in the intrinsic system and the final common pathway of coagulation (Fig. 20.1 on page 126). It is performed by recalcifying citrated plasma in the presence of a 'surface' activator and a 'partial thromboplastin', simulating platelet membrane phospholipid.

A deficiency of a specific coagulation factor (e.g. factor VIII in haemophilia A), a coagulation factor inhibitor, a lupus inhibitor, or inhibition of coagulation by heparin may prolong the APTT. Although it can be prolonged in patients receiving warfarin or those with vitamin K deficiency or severe liver disease, it is less sensitive to these defects than the prothrombin time.

Incorrect specimen collection or handling may result in either a false positive (prolonged) or a false negative (shortened) APTT result (see Table 20.1 on page 126).

In practice, the main uses of the APTT are:

■ monitoring full dose, continuous infusion heparin therapy. For the laboratory's therapeutic interval to be meaningful, the heparin sensitivity of the APTT reagent used must have been established by the laboratory. The APTT has no place in the management of patients receiving low molecular weight heparin or heparinoids.

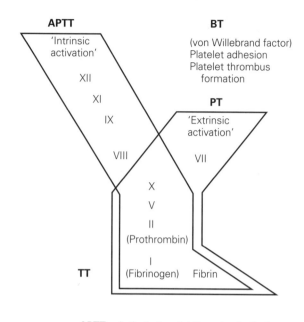

APTT	Activated partial thromboplastin time
BT	Bleeding time
PT	Prothrombin time
TT	Thrombin time

FIGURE 20.1 Basic tests of haemostasis

TABLE 20.1 Causes of an incorrect APTT

Difficult or slow collection
Delay in mixing blood with the citrate anticoagulant
Addition of an incorrect volume of blood to the citrate
Heparin contamination (e.g. in hospital practice, collection in a heparinised syringe or through a heparinised needle)
Prolonged or suboptimal storage of blood before separation of plasma for testing

■ the detection of significant coagulation factor deficiencies in patients with a history suggestive of an inherited bleeding disorder. In the absence of such a clinical history, the yield from the APTT is very low.[2, 3] A normal APTT does not exclude a mild, but clinically significant, coagulation factor deficiency, as most APTT reagents only detect single coagulation factor deficiencies when the level is ≤ 35% of normal. Thus the APTT has little or no value when used as a 'routine' preoperative screening test.

■ the detection of a lupus inhibitor in patients with a history of recurrent foetal loss or recurrent venous and/or arterial thrombosis. Although there are more sensitive screening tests (e.g. the kaolin clotting time, KCT) for the lupus inhibitor, in practice many patients are detected because of a prolongation of the APTT. In spite of sometimes being called the lupus anticoagulant, this antiphospholipid antibody is associated with a tendency to thrombosis, not with a bleeding tendency.

■ the detection of coagulation factor inhibitors (antibodies). Although antibodies to factor VIII or, rarely, factor IX, may develop in haemophilia, they may also occur in patients with autoimmune or lymphoproliferative disorders, in the postpartum period and in previously normal elderly patients. In the non-haemophilia groups, unexplained bleeding of recent onset with an isolated prolongation of the APTT should arouse suspicion that an inhibitor, usually against factor VIII, may be present.

Prothrombin time (PT and INR)

The PT reflects the activity of the 'extrinsic system' and 'final common pathway' of coagulation (Fig. 20.1). It is measured by recalcifying citrated plasma after the addition of a 'complete' thromboplastin (e.g. a suspension of human or animal brain) which simulates tissue factor. Increasingly, thromboplastins produced by recombinant DNA technology are being used for this test. Compared with the APTT, the PT is more sensitive to the coagulation defect induced by oral anticoagulant therapy and less sensitive to the effect of heparin.

In practice, the main uses of the PT are:

■ monitoring oral anticoagulant therapy. For this purpose, the PT result is expressed as an international normalised ratio or INR, which provides a result standardised for local reagents and methodology. The therapeutic interval varies for specific indications and there is currently no consensus in the literature. The North American literature recommends an INR of 2.0–3.5, and specifically an INR of 2.5–3.5 for patients with mechanical prosthetic valves.[4] In Europe, an overall therapeutic interval of 2.5–4.8 is recommended: 3.6–4.8 for patients with mechanical valves.[5] One concern is that some of the differences relate to reagent sensitivity. It has been suggested that an INR of 2.0–3.0 is adequate for the treatment and secondary prevention of venous thromboembolism, and an INR of 2.5–3.5 is appropriate for those with mechanical prosthetic valves, perhaps partly because of the reduced thrombogenicity of modern valves.[6]

- assessing patients with hepatocellular disease. The PT is considered to be a sensitive test of liver function; a prolonged PT, particularly in alcoholic liver disease, is often partly due to concomitant dietary vitamin K deficiency.
- detection of vitamin K deficiency, particularly in the alcoholic, in small bowel malabsorption and after prolonged fasting or vomiting, especially if associated with broad-spectrum antibiotic therapy.

A prolonged PT may be seen in patients with a lupus inhibitor, although the APTT is generally more sensitive. The PT has only a limited role in the assessment of patients with a history suggestive of an inherited bleeding disorder, as factor VII deficiency is rare. As with the APTT, use of the PT as a 'routine' preoperative screening test has little or no value.[2, 3]

Thrombin time (TT)

The thrombin time assesses the conversion of fibrinogen to fibrin and is measured by adding thrombin to citrated plasma. The TT only detects abnormalities of fibrinogen and of fibrin formation (Fig. 20.1).

In practice, the thrombin time is used mainly by the laboratory, rather than as a requested test, to:

- detect heparin in a specimen with an unexplained prolongation of the APTT. A prolonged thrombin time which corrects with protamine sulfate confirms the presence of heparin in the sample.
- assist in the diagnosis of disseminated intravascular coagulation (DIC) in which the thrombin time is prolonged due to the presence of hypofibrinogenaemia and fibrin degradation products (FDP) which interfere with fibrin polymerisation. In DIC, the TT only partially corrects with protamine sulfate.
- detect the rare inherited disorders, hypofibrinogenaemia and afibrinogenaemia.

■ detect dysfibrinogenaemia (an abnormal fibrinogen molecule with abnormal function). Inherited dysfibrinogenaemia is rare, but acquired dysfibrinogenaemia may be seen in patients with hepatocellular carcinoma. A similar functional abnormality may be seen in patients with myeloma, due to the paraprotein interfering with fibrin polymerisation.

Summary

Investigations should address a diagnostic question, rather than being applied as a 'routine'. Provision of an accurate history on the request form and consultation with the pathologist as to appropriate testing should assist the laboratory to answer that question.

REFERENCES

1 Lind S. E. The bleeding time does not predict surgical bleeding [see comments]. *Blood* 1991; 77: 2547–52. Comment in: *Blood* 1992; 79: 2495–7.

2 Eisenberg J. M., Clarke J. R. and Sussman S. A. Prothrombin and partial thromboplastin times as preoperative screening tests. *Arch Surg* 1982; 117: 48–51.

3 Suchman A. L. and Griner P. F. Diagnostic uses of the activated partial thromboplastin time and prothrombin time. *Ann Intern Med* 1986; 104: 810–6.

4 Hirsh J., Dalen J. E., Deykin D. and Poller L. Oral anticoagulants. Mechanism of action, clinical effectiveness, and optimal therapeutic range. *Chest* 1992; 102(4 Suppl): 312S–26S.

5 Loeliger E. A. Therapeutic target values in oral anticoagulation— justification of Dutch policy and a warning against the so-called moderate intensity regimens [published erratum appears in *Ann Hematol* 1992; 64: 253]. *Ann Hematol* 1992; 64: 60–5.

6 Saour J. and Gallus A. Warfarin: is it time to reduce target ranges again? *Aust NZ J Med* 1993; 23: 692–6.

21 | Investigations for thrombotic tendencies

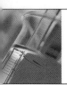

R. Baker

SYNOPSIS

New thrombophilia factors have recently been discovered. They explain the majority of cases of familial or recurrent venous thrombosis and some cases of atherothrombosis. They include activated protein C resistance (Factor V Leiden), prothrombin gene mutation, mild hyperhomocysteinaemia and antiphospholipid antibodies. These factors can identify patients at higher risk of thrombosis who may benefit from prevention and improved treatment strategies. However, these factors are also common in the general population (approximately 1 in 20 people) so a thorough understanding of their significance and clinical management is important.

Introduction

Thrombophilia can be defined as an increased tendency to develop arterial or venous thrombosis which is recurrent, familial, or presents at an unusual site or at a young age. The thrombosis can be catastrophic, leading to death, permanent disability, prolonged periods of hospitalisation or chronic symptoms of lower limb venous insufficiency. The results of appropriate laboratory investigations can help us develop strategies that will either prevent the occurrence of thrombosis or assist with decisions about effective antithrombotic treatment. Until recently, the aetiology of most cases of thrombophilia was largely unknown. This situation has dramatically changed because we now know that over 80% of patients with thrombophilia and venous thrombosis have an abnormality of the natural anticoagulant system.

Clinical assessment is important

Most cases of deep venous thrombosis can be explained by the interaction of plasma coagulation 'thrombophilia' abnormalities and the well-recognised 'clinical' risk factors (such as obesity, major abdominal or orthopaedic surgery, oral contraceptive pill, pregnancy, malignancy or immobility). The larger the number of either clinical or laboratory risk factors, the greater the chance of deep venous thrombosis.

Accurate clinical assessment is important to establish the diagnosis, identify family members at risk, prevent recurrence and rule out other occult disease. Particular emphasis is made on the site and severity of thrombosis, whether or not it occurred spontaneously or postoperatively and if the event is associated with a well-identified precipitating factor such as oestrogen therapy or plane travel. A previously undiagnosed malignancy (particularly a mucin-secreting adenocarcinoma) or a myeloproliferative disorder may present with a similar picture of unusual thrombosis. These conditions should be considered before testing for thrombophilia.

Newly described thrombophilia factors

The frequency and the relative risk of venous thrombosis for the thrombophilia factors are found in Table 21.1 on page 132.[1]

Activated protein C resistance

Activated protein C (APC) resistance is a hereditary defect of the protein C natural anticoagulant pathway (Fig. 21.1). APC normally acts as a natural anticoagulant. It downregulates the intensity of the clotting cascade by neutralising activated coagulation Factor V. This process is inefficient in people with APC resistance. They do not have the crucial APC cleavage site on the Factor V molecule because of a point mutation (Factor V Leiden).

TABLE 21.1 Frequency and relative risk of venous thrombosis for the thrombophilia factors

	PATIENTS WITH DEEP VENOUS THROMBOSIS	GENERAL POPULATION	RELATIVE RISK OF THROMBOSIS
Factor V Leiden	50%	4%	8-fold*
Prothrombin gene mutation	15%	3%	4-fold
Antithrombin III, protein C and S deficiency	10%	1 %	up to 20-fold
Hyperhomocysteinaemia	15%	5%	3-fold
Antiphospholipid antibodies	common	–	8-fold

* risk increased to 35-fold in women on the oral contraceptive pill

This mutation is common, occurring in 4% of randomly selected healthy people in Australia.[2] It can be found in up to 50% of patients with recurrent familial venous thrombosis. The mutation causes an eight-fold increased risk of thrombosis compared to normal. The homozygous form is not infrequent and substantially increases the risk of thrombosis to 100 times normal. The inheritance pattern is autosomal dominant so there is a one in two chance that other family members may have a similar predisposition to thrombosis.[1] APC resistance is usually detected by a sensitive and specific clotting assay and confirmed by molecular analysis for the Factor V Leiden mutation.

Women are especially at risk because oestrogens and pregnancy combined with APC resistance substantially increase the likelihood of thrombosis. The use of a combined oral contraceptive increases the relative risk of thrombosis to 35-fold in those with APC resistance.[3] However, the absolute increased risk for thrombosis is small and is estimated to be 3% over a 10-year period of oral contraceptive use.[1]

In general, APC resistance is not associated with ischaemic heart disease[2] or stroke. However, subgroup analysis reveals a 30-fold increased risk of acute myocardial infarction in young women who smoke or who are obese. There are reports of young women who are homozygous for the Factor V Leiden, presenting with acute myocardial infarction but normal coronary arteries.

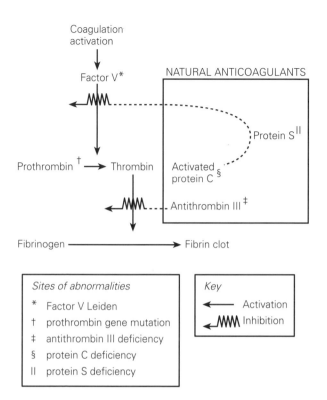

Coagulation
activation

Factor V*

NATURAL ANTICOAGULANTS

Prothrombin † ⟶ Thrombin

Protein S[II]

Activated protein C[§]

Antithrombin III[‡]

Fibrinogen ⟶ Fibrin clot

Sites of abnormalities

* Factor V Leiden
† prothrombin gene mutation
‡ antithrombin III deficiency
§ protein C deficiency
II protein S deficiency

Key

⟵ Activation
⟵〰 Inhibition

FIGURE 21.1 Regulation of coagulation activation and thrombophilia abnormalities

Activation of the blood coagulation system generates large amounts of thrombin which produce cleavage of fibrinogen to form a stable fibrin clot. Natural anticoagulants downregulate the coagulation cascade. Deficiency of these natural anticoagulants, resistant Factor V (Factor V Leiden) and increased prothrombin levels impair downregulation. This predisposes the patient to thrombosis.

Prothrombin gene mutation

A point mutation in the prothrombin molecule causes an increase in its circulating plasma level, predisposing to thrombus formation. The mutation is common in the healthy Australian population (3.3%)[4] and it occurs in up to 15% of patients with thrombophilia. It is estimated to increase the thrombotic risk by four-fold compared to those without the mutation.[1] The mutation can be detected only by DNA polymerase chain reaction (PCR). The inheritance is autosomal dominant.

High homocysteine levels

A high concentration of homocysteine is an independent risk factor for atherothrombosis and venous thrombosis.[5] Although severe hyperhomocysteinaemia is rare, mild hyperhomocysteinaemia is common, occurring in about 5% of the general population, increasing to 15% in patients with venous thrombosis and up to 40% in patients with all forms of premature vascular disease. Mild hyperhomocysteinaemia increases the relative risk of coronary artery disease 24-fold and there is a three-fold increase in the relative risk of venous thrombosis. There appears to be a graded rather than a threshold relationship between plasma homocysteine and the risk of vascular disease and mortality.

Mild elevations of homocysteine concentrations are predominantly caused by a subclinical deficiency of folic acid, vitamin B_{12} or pyridoxine, particularly when also associated with genetic mutations in the enzymes that control the metabolism of methionine (methylene tetrahydrofolate reductase and cystathionine beta synthase). Other causes include chronic renal failure, malignancy, hypothyroidism, cigarette smoking and drugs (methotrexate, phenytoin and theophylline).

Treatment varies with the underlying cause, but correcting vitamin deficiency is generally effective in reducing the homocysteine concentration. Even when there is no detectable vitamin deficiency, folic acid taken in doses of 2–5 mg daily will normalise the homocysteine level. However, randomised clinical trials will be necessary to show that lowering homocysteine levels will have an impact on cardiovascular or thrombotic events. This form of therapy is relatively safe and inexpensive and it would not be unreasonable, while awaiting the results of the prospective clinical trials, to give vitamins to patients with atherothrombosis and hyperhomocysteinaemia.[6]

Antiphospholipid antibodies

Autoantibodies against phospholipid and other molecules on the platelet surface can be associated with atherothrombosis. The antibody type, class, strength and target antigen(s) are extremely varied, not only amongst individual patients but also within the same patient at varying times. The two common laboratory methods used to detect these antibodies are the lupus anticoagulant and the anticardiolipin antibody assays.

The lupus anticoagulants are antiphospholipid antibodies detected by clotting methods. Anticardiolipin antibodies are detected by serological methods. Each of these autoantibodies against phospholipids and other coagulation molecules is associated with both arterial and venous thrombosis. Although most of the time both tests are simultaneously abnormal, only one test may be abnormal in one-third of cases despite identical clinical conditions. These antibodies are common in patients with thrombosis. Their detection is important because there may be a substantial increase in the risk of recurrent thrombosis. However, low titres of autoantibodies are frequently found in the normal population, are of uncertain clinical significance and may be transient, particularly in response to infection.

Prevention of recurrent thrombosis (especially arterial thrombosis) in patients with persistently high antibody titres may require long-term warfarin therapy. This is set at a higher target INR range (3–4.5).[7] Aspirin appears to be less effective in the prevention of recurrent thrombosis than warfarin. Patients with recurrent spontaneous abortions may have antiphospholipid antibodies. The combination of low-dose aspirin (100 mg) and standard heparin (5000 IU twice daily) substantially reduces foetal loss in any subsequent pregnancy. The detection of antiphospholipid antibodies in patients with thrombosis is frequently the only manifestation of the autoimmune disease (known as the primary antiphospholipid antibody syndrome), but it can also be associated with other autoantibody syndromes such as systemic lupus erythematosus.

Coexisting thrombophilia factors increase thrombosis risk

As thrombophilia factors are relatively frequent, compound heterozygotes (such as Factor V Leiden together with the prothrombin gene mutation) are common. This substantially increases the risk of venous thrombosis compared to having only one abnormality[1]. The thrombophilia genes are independently inherited in thrombosis-prone families so they may be absent, or one or other gene may be found, or both abnormalities may coexist. This may explain why in some families the thrombosis phenotype is variable. The risk of thrombosis may be further increased by the coexistence of antiphospholipid antibodies or high levels of homocysteine.

Technical aspects
Laboratory testing

A diagnosis of thrombophilia should ensure appropriate prophylaxis is given in high-risk situations such as after surgery, immobility, long plane flights, during pregnancy and postpartum. Prevention includes measures such as anticoagulant therapy (standard heparin or low molecular weight heparin), early mobilisation and increasing lower limb venous blood flow (compression stocking and plantar plexus foot pump). The intensity of prophylaxis against venous thrombosis depends on the perceived hazard in each case versus the risk reduction by intervention. At the very least, diagnosis of a thrombophilia factor should ensure preventive measures are considered even in family members without a history of thrombosis.

Who to test?

Any patient with spontaneous, unusual, recurrent or a strong family history of venous thrombosis or evidence of premature arterial occlusion should be tested. It is reasonable to test first-degree relatives for an identified hereditary thrombophilia factor because half the family members will inherit the mutation. Finding the abnormality will provide an opportunity to modify other risk factors and ensure appropriate prophylaxis against venous thrombosis in high-risk situations.

Which test and when?

Patients can be tested (Table 21.2) either at the presentation of thrombosis or after finishing anticoagulation. Abnormal results should always be confirmed by repeat testing. This is because the levels of the natural anticoagulant factors may be altered by consumption in the clotting process, blood collection artefacts and standardisation and reproducibility problems inherent in most of the clotting-based laboratory techniques. Testing other family members without thrombosis to confirm the hereditary nature of

TABLE 21.2 Suggested laboratory tests for thrombophilia*—consultation with the pathology laboratory is recommended

Full blood examination and erythrocyte sedimentation rate†
Factor V Leiden (activated protein C resistance)
Plasma homocysteine
Prothrombin gene mutation
Anticardiolipin antibodies
Lupus anticoagulant
Antithrombin III
Protein C, protein S‡

---

* The Medicare rebate is at present approximately $145. There is currently no rebate for the DNA testing for Factor V Leiden and the prothrombin gene mutation. Around 25 mL of blood is required. All tests can be performed when the patient is on heparin.

† Examines for myeloproliferative disorders and occult systemic diseases

‡ Should only be done before (or 2 weeks after ceasing) oral anticoagulation

the problem is often helpful for a patient with uncertain results due to acute thrombosis or anticoagulation.

Molecular confirmation of the Factor V Leiden mutation is recommended not only to confirm the abnormal clotting result, but also to differentiate clearly a homozygote and heterozygote carrier. Protein C and S are vitamin K-dependent anticoagulant factors and so deficiency cannot be diagnosed while the patient is on warfarin. However, all the thrombophilia factors can usually be tested while the patient is on therapeutic heparin or low molecular weight heparin. Routine homocysteine testing is only now entering clinical practice and it is uncertain if fasting levels or a methionine load test (analogous to a glucose tolerance test for diabetes) will be required.

Summary

Thrombophilia factors are frequently found in the majority of patients with recurrent or familial venous thrombosis. Obtaining a familial history of thrombosis is now analogous to a bleeding history (particularly if the patient has a convincing family history of deep venous thrombosis and is considering surgery or the oral contraceptive pill). Laboratory testing can be used to see if these patients have a higher risk of thrombosis. This information leads to better informed choices and the development of strategies to prevent thrombosis. However, most patients with these thrombophilia factors will never develop thrombosis in their lifetime. The occurrence of thrombosis is explained in people who are at high risk because of the accumulation of an increasing number of either clinical and/or thrombophilia factors.

REFERENCES

1 Rosendaal F. R. Risk factors for venous thrombosis: prevalence, risk and interaction. *Semin Hematol* 1997; 34: 171–87.

2 van Bockxmeer F. M., Baker R. I. and Taylor R. R. Premature ischaemic heart disease and the gene for coagulation factor V [letter]. *Nat Med* 1995; 1: 185.

3 Vandenbroucke J. P., Koster T., Briet E., Reitsma P. H., Bertina R. M. and Rosendaal F. R. Increased risk of venous thrombosis in oral contraceptive users who are carriers of the Factor V Leiden mutation. *Lancet* 1994; 344: 1453–7.

4 Eikelboom J. W., Baker R. I., Parsons R., Taylor R. R. and van Bockxmeer F. M. No association between the 20210 G/A prothrombin gene mutation and premature coronary artery disease. *Thromb Haemost* 1998; 80: 878–80.

5 Welch G. N. and Loscalzo J. Homocysteine and atherothrombosis. *N Engl J Med* 1998; 338: 1042–50.

6 Wilcken D. E. Homocysteine and vascular disease [editorial]. *Med J Aust* 1998; 168: 431–2.

7 Khamashta M. A., Cuadrado M. J., Mujic F., Taub N. A., Hunt B. J. and Hughes G. R. The management of thrombosis in the antiphospholipid-antibody syndrome. *N Engl J Med* 1995; 332: 993–7.

Urine testing

J. F. Mahony

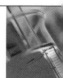

Introduction

Urine is tested to determine the presence or otherwise of urinary tract disease. Macroscopic examination, a 'dip-stick' test, microscopy and culture of appropriately collected fresh urine are the usual methods. Repeated fixed abnormalities may lead to specific diagnosis. Normal urine is rare in patients with progressive renal disease; the exceptions are renovascular disease and interstitial nephritis.

Technical aspects

A standard method of urine collection

The midstream urine is best collected in the following sequence:

1 Wash hands
2 Expose and wash external genitalia with dilute soap solution and rinse with sterile water using pads or cotton-wool balls. *Do not use antiseptics.*
3 Pass a small amount of urine.
4 Collect the next aliquot into a wide-mouthed sterile container.
5 Cap and label.

- All urine should be examined fresh, preferably using an early morning or concentrated specimen.
- Each specimen should be collected as a midstream specimen.
- Examination of a centrifuged deposit, 5 minutes at 3000 rpm, improves the detection of casts and crystals.
- There is considerable inter-laboratory variation in reception, handling and reporting of urine tests.
- Mechanical means of counting cells and casts in urine have recently proved useful and will play a greater role in future.

Is the result abnormal?

One or more of the following abnormalities may be found in asymptomatic patients. Often the presence of two such abnormalities allows a confident diagnosis.

Macroscopic examination

Red urine may be due to the presence of blood, beetroot or rifampicin. Dark-brown urine may be due to porphyrins, old blood and alkaptonuria. Rarely, melanoma can cause black urine. Cloudy urine is usually due to phosphates and frothy urine to proteinuria. A milky appearance and high fat content can be due to chyluria, usually seen in filariasis and, less often, lymphatic obstruction.

Urinalysis

Proteinuria

Commercially available test strips are specific for albumin and microalbumin. They do not detect protein in normal urine, or Bence Jones protein. False positives may, however, occur and 'trace' findings should usually be disregarded. Proteinuria should be quantitated and confirmed with other tests (e.g. sulfonylsalicylic acid, which detects all proteins and not only albumin). In young people, postural (orthostatic) proteinuria should be excluded. Persistent proteinuria requires investigation and 24-hour urinary protein is the first test.

Microalbuminuria

Commercial test strips are now available to detect and measure small amounts of albumin, at 0, 20, 50 and 100 mg/L. The detection of microalbumin in patients with diabetes mellitus is critical for the identification of those at risk of progressive diabetic nephropathy.

Haematuria

Dip-sticks are quite sensitive. Positives should be confirmed microscopically and red cell casts sought in a centrifuged deposit. Even if the patient is asymptomatic, full investigation of renal function and urinary tracts is mandatory—some 80% of older patients will have urological causes, including carcinoma, prostatic hypertrophy in men and urethrotrigonitis in women. Usually good quality renal ultrasound and cystoscopy are both necessary to exclude malignancy. Even if normal, careful follow-up for at least 2 years is advised. Myoglobin can also react with Haemostix, so should be considered (and confirmed spectroscopically) when red cells are not seen microscopically; elevated serum muscle enzyme levels also implicate myoglobin.

Glycosuria

Investigate for diabetes mellitus or renal glycosuria.

Urinary pH

Urinary pH is useful in some forms of management. Diagnostically, persistently alkaline urine may indicate stones, renal tubular acidosis, or infection due to *Proteus* sp. Persistently acid urine may indicate gout.

Specific gravity (SG)

SG must be interpreted in the context of the timing of urine collection, state of hydration, recent fluid intake, recent intravenous pyelogram, and so on. If SG is 1.010 under varying conditions, advanced renal failure is likely. The SG allows a better interpretation of proteinuria; for instance, trace proteinuria with SG 1.030 (concentrated urine) is unlikely to be of any significance.

Microscopic examination of urine

White cells

Normal urine contains less than 2000 leucocytes per millilitre. Pyuria is most often due to urinary tract infection; sterile pyuria may be found in analgesic nephropathy, calculus disease, gonococcal urethritis, tuberculosis, partially treated infection or, most often, a poor urine collection. The presence of numerous epithelial cells also indicates poor technique in collection. Persistent sterile pyuria is an indication for intravenous pyelography and further early morning collections for detection and culture of acid-fast bacilli.

TABLE 22.1 Normal urine

PROPERTY	AMOUNT	COMMENTS
SG	1000–1030	Depends on hydration—fixed 1010 indicates renal disease
pH	5–8	Usually acid in morning
Protein	0–trace	Especially in concentrated urine, alkaline urine
Blood	0	Avoid menstrual urinalysis; a very sensitive test
Glucose	0	Positive in diabetes mellitus/renal glycosuria
Microalbumin	0	First sign of diabetic nephropathy
WCC	< 2000/mL	Consider sterile pyuria if negative culture
RBC	< 1000/mL	Consider myoglobin if positive dipstick
Bacteria	< 10^4	Depends on site of urine
Hyaline	+	In concentrated urine

Red cells
Red cells are rare in normal urine; more than 1000 per millilitre or more than 2 per high power field are abnormal and require investigation. Finding significant proteinuria or red cell casts in the same urine indicates a primary glomerular or systemic vascular lesion. Microscopic haematuria in the presence of pyuria is likely to be due to trigonitis or other lower urinary tract infection. The percentage of dysmorphic red cells, if greater than 80%, may help differentiate 'glomerular' causes from lower tract causes of bleeding.

Casts
Casts are likely to be formed when urinary protein excretion is increased and/or flow rate is low.

Hyaline casts

Hyaline casts are found in normal concentrated urine and require no further investigation.

White cell casts

White cell casts indicate that infection is present and likely to be of renal origin; in a male, or in a female with recurrent infection, further investigation is always justified.

Red cell casts

Red cell casts are significant in that glomerular injury due to glomerulonephritis, severe hypertension or vasculitis is responsible; further investigations aimed at determining the presence of an antigen (antistreptolysin O titre, DNA antibody binding activity, hepatitis B surface antigen, hepatitis C antibody, and so on) or activation of immune complexes (cryoglobulins, immunoglobulins etc.) should precede renal biopsy.

Granular casts

Granular casts and haem casts probably have the same origin and significance as red cell casts.

Broad casts

Broad casts indicate the tubular atrophy and interstitial fibrosis of chronic renal failure, but are uncommon. Serum electrolytes, creatinine and urea nitrogen will reveal the degree and consequences of renal impairment.

Crystals

Crystals are commonly seen in the urinary sediment, best found in warm (37°C) specimens, but are not often useful in the detection of renal disorders. In asymptomatic individuals, calcium oxalate crystals are found more often than uric acid or other crystals. Both calcium oxalate and uric acid crystals may be found in 'normals' with acid urine, with a diet high in oxalates and purines respectively, and when the urine is concentrated; however, both may also be found in stone formers, and uric acid in gout or treated lymphomas. Cystine crystals are rare, being found in cystinuria and other related aminoacidurias.

Bacteriuria and cultures

Bacteria

Bacteria are never seen in fresh and properly collected normal urine. Their presence in fresh urine indicates significant urinary tract infection. Normal midstream urine contains less than 1000 organisms per mL after culture; more than 10^5 per mL of a single organism usually indicate bacterial infection; and any organisms are significant in a suprapubic specimen in a child. Between 10^4 and 10^5 organisms per mL are regarded as equivocal, requiring a repeat test but, if found in a clinical setting such as indwelling catheter, renal calculus or diabetes mellitus, infection is likely. Mixed cultures of two organisms may also be found in the above settings but are more often due to contamination from using a poor collection technique. One should be suspicious of a report of bacteriuria when pus cells are absent from urine; the usual causes are a poor collection technique (indicated by the presence of many epithelial cells) or a prolonged delay in examining the urine after its collection. The test should be repeated with careful attention to the collection technique (see box, *A standard method of urine collection*) before initiating antibacterial therapy in an asymptomatic patient. Repeated cultures of the same organism suggest renal rather than lower urinary tract infection.

The organism identified by culture must also be considered. The usual pathogens are *E. coli*, other coliforms, *Streptococcus faecalis* and *Klebsiella*; *Proteus* and *Pseudomonas* ssp. are also found, especially in patients with calculi. *Staphylococcus epidermidis* and *Staphylococcus aureus* are occasionally pathogenic. Well-recognised contaminants include skin organisms such as *Staphylococcus epidermidis*, and normal vaginal flora such as diphtheroids; on rare occasions such bacteria and pyuria are found in properly collected urine on two occasions and require treatment.

Drug sensitivities

Antibacterial agents which are well concentrated in urine are most often used and sensitivities to sulfonamides, trimethoprim, nitrofurantoin, nalidixic acid, ampicillin, tetracycline, cephalosporins, norfloxacin and aminoglycoside antibiotics are usually reported. Such a range is necessary to allow for variations in the sensitivities of organisms to the drugs, patient allergy, age, pregnancy and/or renal impairment. Occasionally, further drug sensitivities are required, particularly when infection is chronic, e.g. when there is an indwelling catheter.

Antibacterial activity
The presence of antibacterial activity will explain sterile pyuria or failure to show a positive culture in suspicious clinical circumstances.

Combinations

Proteinuria and haematuria
Proteinuria and haematuria are hallmarks of glomerulonephritis, especially when proteinuria is severe. However, both may be found in 'normals' after jogging or heavy exercise, as well as in urinary tract infection, neoplasm and hypertension. Finding red cell casts makes lower-tract pathology unlikely and investigation is directed towards renal parenchymal disease. The urine should be retested at least 48 hours later in people who go jogging.

Haematuria
Haematuria and infection are most likely due to urethrotrigonitis in women and prostatitis in men.

Red cells, white cells, casts
Red cells, white cells, casts of both and eosinophils are seen in interstitial nephritis, most commonly due to drugs including methicillin and other penicillins, and sulphonamides.

A sediment of red cells, white cells, red cell or granular casts, broad casts and lipiduria
These indicate a severe glomerular lesion with a nephrotic element and are most often seen in collagen disorders such as systemic lupus erythematosus.

FURTHER READING

Gyory A. Z. et al. Clinical value of urine microscopy by normal and automated methods. *Lab Hematology* 1998; 4: 211–6.

Schroder F. H. Microscopic haematuria requires investigation. *Br Med J* 1994; 309: 70–2.

Yamagata K. et al. A long-term follow-up study of asymptomatic haematuria and/or proteinuria in adults. *Clin Neph* 1996; 45: 281–8.

23 | Hepatitis B testing

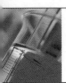

S. Nicholson and I. Gust

Introduction

The laboratory diagnosis of hepatitis B viral (HBV) infection is achieved by identification of HBV-associated antigens and antibodies in the blood. To distinguish between acute and chronic infection, to determine immune status or evaluate viral replication it is necessary to test for particular serological markers.

Hepatitis B virus structure and antigens

The hepatitis B virus (HBV) (or Dane particle) is a 42-nanometre spherical particle consisting of an outer shell of hepatitis B surface antigen (Australia antigen) (HBsAg) and an inner core containing a second antigen (HBcAg), which encloses a single molecule of circular, partially double-stranded DNA and a DNA polymerase. Another antigen, HBeAg, is secreted from hepatocytes directly into blood as a soluble protein.[1] The blood of infected individuals contains not only mature virions but large numbers of spherical particles (22 nanometres) and tubules (22 nanometres x 100–150 nanometres) which are composed of excess HBsAg. While HBsAg and HBeAg are directly detectable in the serum, HBcAg is usually not. During infection, the patient may produce an antibody response with development of anti-HBs, anti-HBc and anti-HBe, which can be detected in the serum.

Serum markers of hepatitis B infection

Infection with HBV is acquired by contact with blood or body secretions. The incubation period is usually about 3 months, but can range from 40 to 180 days.

The majority of individuals infected with hepatitis B experience a transient subclinical infection which is followed by clearance of the virus and production of antibody. Approximately one-third of infected individuals develop acute hepatitis that may be severe enough to require hospitalisation and some 90% of infected infants and 5–10% of adults become chronic carriers of hepatitis B virus after symptomatic or asymptomatic infection. When infection occurs early in life and is followed by chronic carriage of the virus, an increased incidence of chronic persistent hepatitis, chronic active hepatitis (with or without cirrhosis) and primary hepatocellular carcinoma may occur. The high chronic carrier rate in infants has led to the development of an infant vaccination program.

Acute

During the incubation period, HBsAg appears in the blood; in this early period, active viral replication is taking place so HBeAg, HBV DNA and DNA polymerase are also detectable. DNA polymerase is not tested for in the diagnostic laboratory, however. Peak levels of virus markers are usually reached about the time that symptoms appear and serum aminotransferase levels are peaking. In uncomplicated infections, levels of HBsAg begin to decline and usually fall to undetectable levels within 3 months of the onset of illness. A decline in HBsAg is accompanied by a loss of other markers of viral replication (HBeAg, HBV DNA and DNA polymerase) and the appearance of viral antibodies—specifically anti-HBc, anti-HBe and anti-HBs. (See Fig. 23.1 on page 148.)

Anti-HBc appears just before or at the onset of illness. Initially, most of the antibody is of the IgM class, but, as time passes, the IgM titre decreases while the IgG level increases. These antibodies persist for many years.

The second antibody to appear is anti-HBe, usually about the time that HBeAg becomes undetectable. This antibody does not normally reach high levels and disappears within a few months or years.

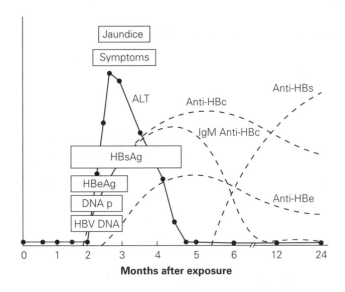

FIGURE 23.1 The typical serological course of an acute type B hepatitis infection

Reprinted with permission from *Perspectives on Viral Hepatitis*, 1981, p. 6, courtesy of Abbott Diagnostics.

The last antibody to appear is anti-HBs which may not become detectable for 3–6 months after the onset of illness. Anti-HBs persists for years, although the titre decreases with time. In a large proportion of patients, there is often a period after HBsAg has disappeared and before anti-HBs has appeared; during this gap, which can be weeks or months, the only detectable marker of recent HBV infection may be the presence of anti-HBc IgM. In a small percentage of patients, anti-HBs is not produced or is produced in very low levels, even though HBsAg has been cleared and the patient has recovered.

There are also a number of variations on this serological profile.

Chronic

Persistence of HBsAg for more than 6 months indicates that the patient has become a chronic carrier of the virus. The serological pattern in chronic infection depends upon the degree of activity of the virus. In a patient who has been recently infected and has just become a chronic carrier, markers of active replication (HBeAg, HBV DNA and DNA polymerase) are likely to be present, in which case the anti-HBc response is mainly IgM. The anti-HBc IgM response usually decreases to low levels or becomes undetectable in the chronic carrier. However, there may be periods of active viral replication whereby 'spikes' (sharp increase in levels) of anti-HBc IgM may appear. Other carriers in which replication is occurring at a relatively low rate have no markers of active replication or very low levels of HBV DNA, and HBeAg is replaced by anti-HBe. (See Fig. 23.2.)

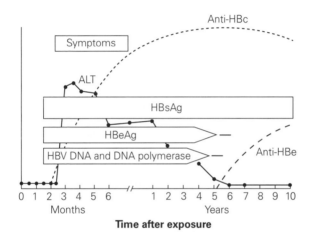

Time after exposure

FIGURE 23.2 The clinical, serological and biochemical course of a chronic type B hepatitis infection

Reprinted with permission from *Perspectives on Viral Hepatitis*, 1981, p. 8, courtesy of Abbott Diagnostics.

Between 0.5% and 2.5% of chronic carriers per annum eventually clear HBsAg; this is largely attributable to clearance of viremia.[2]

Technical aspects

The diagnosis of HBV infection is achieved by identification of HBV-associated antigens and antibodies in blood. This is achieved by using sensitive tests such as enzyme-linked immunosorbent assays (ELISAs) or microparticle enzyme immunoassay (MEIAs). For evaluation of viral replication, molecular hybridisation tests or polymerase chain reaction (PCR) for HBV DNA are used.

Results for antigen and antibody levels are reported as either negative or positive. With anti-HBs results, an indication of the amount of antibody detected is given by a signal to noise ratio (S/N) or mIU/mL. An S/N or mIU/mL greater than 10 is usually defined as a protective level of antibody.

Summary of serological markers for HBV infection

- *Hepatitis B surface antigen* (HBsAg)—first marker to appear in acute infection; persists in chronic infection which is defined by two positive HBsAg results 6 months apart.
- *Hepatitis Be antigen* (HBeAg)—appears early in active acute infection (at the same time or shortly after HBsAg). Its presence indicates active replication and high infectivity in either acute or chronic infection. It is usually short-lived (2–8 weeks in acute infection); persistence beyond 12 weeks suggests progression to the chronic carrier state.
- *Hepatitis B core antibody* (anti-HBc)—early indicator of acute infection; initially most of the antibody is of the IgM class, but as time passes, the IgM titre decreases while the IgG level increases; in chronic infection, low levels of anti-HBc IgM may persist. Anti-HBc persists for life and is a useful marker of current or past infection. Anti-HBc IgM may be useful in confirming a diagnosis of acute hepatitis B, especially in the 'window' phase when HBsAg has disappeared and anti-HBs is not yet detectable.
- *Hepatitis Be antibody* (anti-HBe)—appears in acute and chronic infection as the infection is resolving.
- *Hepatitis B surface antibody* (anti-HBs)—marker of clinical recovery and immunity to hepatitis B virus. Used to determine the immune status of hepatitis B vaccinated individuals.
- *HBV DNA*—presence in the serum indicates active viral replication and high infectivity; may be detected when HBeAg is absent or in low levels. Detectable HBV DNA levels persisting longer than 8 weeks may be indicative of progressing to the chronic carrier state.

Summary of most useful markers for diagnosis

Table 23.1 summarises the most useful markers for diagnosis.

TABLE 23.1 The most useful markers for diagnosis

Acute infection	HBsAg, anti-HBc IgM
Chronic infection	HBsAg, anti-HBc IgM
Infectivity	(if patient is HBsAg positive)
	HBV DNA, HBeAg, anti-HBe
Current or past infection	anti-HBc
Immunity	anti-HBs

REFERENCES

1 Siebert D. and Locarnini S. Hepatitis B issues in laboratory diagnosis and vaccination. *Aust Prescr* 1998; 21(3): 72–5.

2 Kato Y., Nakao K., Hamasaki K., Kato H., Nakata K., Kusumoto Y. and Eguchi K. Spontaneous loss of hepatitis B surface antigen in chronic carriers, based on a long-term follow-up study in Goto Islands, Japan. *J. Gastroenterol* 2000; 35(3): 201–5.

24 | Hepatitis B: issues in laboratory diagnosis and vaccination

D. Siebert and S. Locarnini

SYNOPSIS

A laboratory diagnosis of hepatitis B (HBV) infection depends on the detection of hepatitis B surface antigen in serum. The distinction between acute and chronic infection relies on the detection of other serological markers. Serum-based assays can now detect and quantify the viral DNA. These assays will have a role in therapeutic monitoring and the detection of HBV mutants.

While new guidelines for vaccination have recently been published, some issues regarding revaccination and the management of people who cannot mount an adequate vaccine response are yet to be adequately resolved.

Introduction

In Australia, almost 1% of the population may be chronically infected with hepatitis B virus (HBV). This results in up to 1200 deaths annually.[1] The highest carriage rates are in indigenous people (10–25%), Micronesian and South-East Asian immigrants (5–15%) and people from South-East Europe (2–5%). Despite the existence of an established maternal screening and infant vaccination program, it has been virtually impossible to identify people at risk before their exposure to the virus. Vaccination aimed at high-risk groups has therefore failed to significantly reduce the burden of chronic infection in low prevalence countries like Australia.[1] For these reasons, a new program of universal vaccination has recently been recommended.[2]

Viral structure and products

Hepatitis B virus is a compact, 42 nm sphere (Fig. 24.1). The outer envelope is composed of units made from hepatitis B surface antigen (HBsAg) proteins, carbohydrates and lipids. Beneath this outer layer is found the core, a 27 nm particle, made of protein subunits called hepatitis B core antigen (HBcAg).

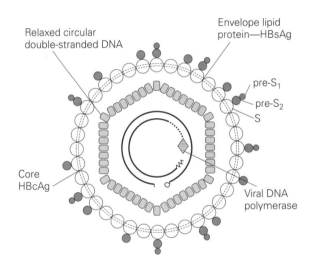

FIGURE 24.1 A model of hepatitis B virus—note the three components of surface antigen: pre-S$_1$, pre-S$_2$ and S

The hepatitis Be antigen (HBeAg) is not a structural molecule; however, more than two-thirds of its amino acid sequence is identical to that of the core protein. It can be secreted from hepatocytes directly into blood as a soluble protein,[3] which is thought to promote and maintain persistent infection.

Acute hepatitis B infection

HBV is acquired by contact with blood or body fluids containing infectious virus. Infectivity has been clearly shown only for blood, genital secretions and, on occasion, saliva. The incubation period ranges from 6 to 26 weeks with an average of 12 weeks (Fig. 24.2).

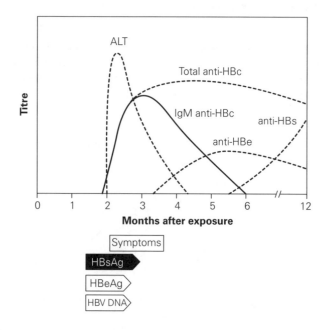

FIGURE 24.2 A graphic representation of serological events in acute hepatitis B. Major markers, hepatitis B surface antigen (HBsAg) and anti-hepatitis B core IgM (anti-HBc IgM) are in bold.
ALT = alanine aminotransferase; total anti-HBc = anti-HBc IgM + IgG

Laboratory diagnosis

HBsAg first appears in the blood during the incubation period while the virus is actively 'replicating' in liver cells. The antigen is produced in vast excess so that it is not only associated with new infectious virus particles, but also occurs in the serum as small non-infectious spherical and filamentous forms. In acute infection, the HBsAg usually disappears within 3 months of onset. The

HBeAg and HBV DNA can also be detected in blood while the virus is actively replicating in the liver (Fig. 24.2). Symptoms usually appear as the concentrations of bilirubin, alanine aminotransferase and each of the major viral components peak in the serum. These events coincide with the first appearance of antibodies to HBV proteins (Fig. 24.2). (See Table 24.1.)

TABLE 24.1 Primary markers for the diagnosis of acute hepatitis B infection

	HBV antigens		Anti-HBV antibodies				
	HBsAg	HBeAg			Ant HBc	Ant HBe	Anti-Hbs
Diagnosis	HBsAg	HBeAg	HBV DNA	IgM	Total Ig		
Acute HBV	++	+	+	++	+	−	−
Resolving							
early	−	±	+	±	±	±	±
late	−	−	−	−	+	+	+
Immune							
vaccination	−	−	−	−	−	−	+
past infection	−	−	−	−	+	−	+

Antibody to HBcAg (anti-HBc) rises first. As a generalisation, the detection of IgM antibody specific to the hepatitis B core is the primary indicator of acute infection. It usually appears at or just before the onset of symptoms and remains detectable for at least 6 months. The IgG component of anti-HBc usually persists for life.

Anti-HBe is the second antibody to appear and is associated with the rapid clearance of HBeAg. Later, anti-HBe declines and persists for only a few months or years if there is no active viral replication.

The antibody to HBsAg, anti-HBs, may not become detectable for 3–6 months after acute infection. It is associated with resolution of the illness. This antibody is recognised as the marker of immunity to HBV.

There is a range of variations in the serological profile and when in doubt an expert opinion can be sought. For example, in some patients who clear HBsAg and recover clinically, the anti-HBs antibody may be present only at low levels or remains below the level of detection.

Chronic hepatitis B infection

Between 1% and 10% of infected adults and older children develop chronic infection. Adults who develop chronic HBV are not usually immunosuppressed but, when they are, chronic infection is common. More than 85–95% of newborns and children infected under the age of 3 years, born to HBeAg positive mothers, become chronic carriers. This is thought to occur because of the immunological immaturity in the child and the effect of maternal HBeAg in utero. Those carriers infected in early life have an increased risk of both chronic persistent and chronic active hepatitis.

Laboratory diagnosis

From a laboratory perspective, chronic infection is defined as the persistence of HBsAg in the blood for a period of 6 months or more. The serological picture depends on the degree of viral activity in chronically infected hepatocytes (Fig. 24.3). (See Table 24.2.)

A recently infected chronic carrier will show evidence of ongoing viral replication in liver cells. HBeAg and HBV DNA can be detected in blood for months or years after acute infection. High levels of anti-HBc IgM antibody are no longer present.

People with long-standing HBV infection may eventually enter a phase of low level viral replication. To achieve this, chronic carriers must clear HBeAg and HBV DNA from the blood by actively producing anti-HBe antibody and clearing viral DNA from infected liver cells, mostly via cell-mediated immunity.[3] Several abortive attempts to clear HBeAg may occur over many years and 'flares' of active hepatitis can occur (with or without symptoms) until anti-HBe is eventually made (Fig. 24.3). Patients who cannot clear the virus face persistent active hepatitis and are at a very high risk for the development of cirrhosis and hepatocellular carcinoma.

HBe antigen negative chronic hepatitis B

Unfortunately, there are exceptions to these principles. Some people, especially those who acquire HBV in very early life, never fully clear HBV from the blood. Due to the pressure of the host's immune system, mutant forms of the HBV can be selected from the pool of infected liver cells. HBV DNA production may continue, despite the absence of HBeAg and the presence of anti-HBe in up to 30% of patients infected early in life (Fig. 24.3).

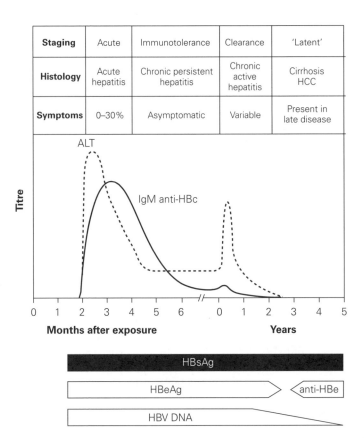

Staging	Acute	Immunotolerance	Clearance	'Latent'
Histology	Acute hepatitis	Chronic persistent hepatitis	Chronic active hepatitis	Cirrhosis HCC
Symptoms	0–30%	Asymptomatic	Variable	Present in late disease

FIGURE 24.3 A graphic representation of the clinical, histological and serological events during chronic hepatitis B in adults.
ALT = alanine aminotransferase

TABLE 24.2 Primary markers for the diagnosis of chronic hepatitis B infection

	HBV antigens			Anti-HBV antibodies			
	HBsAg	HBeAg			Anti-HBc	Anti-HBe	Anti-HBs
Diagnosis			HBV DNA	IgM	Total Ig		
HBeAg positive Chronic hepatitis B	+	+	++		++	–	–
HBeAg negative Chronic hepatitis B	+	–	+/++		++	±	–

Testing patients for hepatitis B in practice

The most commonly used tests are enzyme immunoassays (EIA) for the detection of viral proteins and antibodies. HBV DNA can be quantified by molecular hybridisation assay, and polymerase chain reaction (PCR) tests can detect minute quantities of HBV DNA in serum.

The results for HBsAg are reported as positive or negative. A positive result indicates either acute or chronic infection.

Hepatitis B specific core IgM results are also reported as either positive or negative. In general, a positive result indicates recent infection.

In chronic infection HBsAg is still present, but anti-HBc IgM has disappeared in all but a few patients with 'chronic active' hepatitis. Patients who are positive for HBeAg and/or HBV DNA in the blood are highly infectious carriers. Patients with very low levels of HBV DNA in the blood, usually in the presence of anti-HBe as well, are inactive carriers with low infectivity (Table 24.2).

Between 10% and 20% of chronic carriers eventually clear HBsAg. Like patients recovering from acute infection, they produce anti-HBs antibody. Convalescent patients usually have IgG antibodies to both HBsAg and HBcAg. Vaccinated patients have only antibodies to HBsAg (Table 24.1). The titre of anti-HBs is usually expressed as IU/mL of blood. A titre of 10 IU/mL is the minimum standard for protective immunity to HBV.

Vaccination and revaccination for hepatitis B

Vaccination against HBV was introduced to control the morbidity and mortality associated with the virus. Until 1997, most Western countries, including Australia, had policies aimed at limiting the spread of the virus only in at-risk individuals, rather than population-based immunisation strategies (i.e. universal infant immunisation with a catch-up program). As part of the World Health Organization (WHO) program for the control of hepatitis B, this selective policy has now been abandoned and a wider program adopted.[2, 4]

Until HBV can be incorporated into multivalent childhood vaccines, all adolescents between 10 and 16 years who have not previously been vaccinated should receive 3 doses of standard HBV vaccine. At-risk infants, those with a HBsAg positive mother or those from high prevalence (>2%) communities (e.g. Aboriginal and Torres Strait Islanders, migrants from Africa, Oceania and other endemic areas) should start a course of 3 vaccinations within 7 days of birth. In addition to the vaccine, the children of HBsAg-positive mothers should receive 100 IU hepatitis B immune globulin (HBIG) intramuscularly into the lateral thigh within 12 hours of birth.

Occupational risk groups and other at-risk adults should also be considered for HBV vaccination according to the new NHMRC guidelines (Table 24.3).[2]

TABLE 24.3 Individuals at increased risk of acquiring HBV infection who should be routinely vaccinated—NHMRC guidelines, 2000[2]

Newborns of carrier mothers
Children under 10 years in high (> 2%) prevalence communities
Household contacts of acute and chronic hepatitis B carriers (excluding sexual partners)
People at risk of sexual transmission
Injecting drug users
Haemodialysis patients (often poor vaccine responders)
Blood concentrate recipients
Persons with chronic liver disease/hepatitis C
Residents and staff of facilities for the intellectually disabled
Close contacts of deinstitutionalised people with intellectual disabilities
Long-term prison inmates and staff of correctional facilities
Healthcare workers and embalmers
Others (e.g. day care personnel, police, armed forces personnel, long-stay travellers to endemic countries—see the guidelines)

Revaccination

Most people who seroconvert to the vaccine develop antibody titres greater than 100 I/U/mL within 6–8 weeks of completing the schedule. The antibody response in adults is generally detectable for longer than 11 years and can exceed 15 years in children. The NHMRC advises that booster doses are no longer required for immunocompetent people. [2, 4]

Approximately 5–15% of healthy immunocompetent individuals either fail to mount an antibody response (they are 'non-responders') and remain at risk of infection or respond poorly to the vaccine (these people were previously known as 'hypo-responders').

Vaccine non-responders

A non-responder is a person who, despite a correctly administered full course of standard vaccine, does not mount an anti-HBs response when tested 8–12 weeks after the third vaccination. An anti-HBs titre of less than 1·0 IU/mL indicates a failure to respond to vaccination. Occasionally failure to respond to HBV vaccine is due to HBV infection itself. For at-risk patients, a check for HBsAg and anti-HBc can avoid a delayed diagnosis.

Pre-exposure prophylaxis in non-responders

One strategy for dealing with non-responders is to first evaluate the risk to the individual patient and then re-treat only those at risk. If the patient has no identifiable risk factors for HBV and does not work in an environment that places them at high risk of HBV transmission, then revaccination is not essential. However, those who do have an identifiable risk factor (such as surgeons and dentists) should receive training in standard precautions and risk reduction. In addition, a fourth double-dose or a course of three further injections, spaced at monthly intervals, will succeed in a number of at-risk patients. When using the latter schedule, the vaccinee should be checked for seroconversion 2 weeks after each additional dose.

The next generation of vaccines is likely to incorporate pre-S_1 and pre-S_2 components of HBsAg (Fig. 24.1). One partially controlled trial of a candidate vaccine has shown seroconversion in 70% of non-responders after a single dose of vaccine.[5] Such vaccines may become available in the next few years.

Post-exposure prophylaxis in non-responders

Any individual who has not responded to HBV vaccination and later has an identifiable or high-risk exposure to HBV (e.g. needle-stick injury), should be offered HBIG within 72 hours of exposure. A course of HBV vaccine should also commence within 7 days. While some individuals will have a response to this vaccination, others will be at risk of acute or chronic infection until better vaccines become available. There is as yet no role for antiviral drug prophylaxis but it may be an option in the future, after appropriate trials.

Hypo-responders

In the past, in the U.K. and parts of Europe, a healthy vaccinee who developed an anti-HBs titre of greater than 100 IU/mL was deemed a hypo-responder and was considered to be at risk of HBV infection. This classification is no longer in use.[4] Recent data from Europe and the U.S.A. indicate that any significant response to HBV vaccine in an immunocompetent individual protects against breakthrough infection.[4, 6] Except for the immunocompromised, booster dosing is no longer considered necessary in hypo-responders.[4]

In general, it is considered beneficial to revaccinate high-risk immunocompromised patients in a number of different clinical settings.[2, 4] The practice of any one organisation will be based on the local frequency, type and degree of exposure to HBV as well as the level of immunocompromise. Consultation with an infectious disease physician or a medical virologist is advisable when constructing a vaccination program for high-risk patients, including those with chronic renal failure, transplanted organs or HIV infection.

REFERENCES

1 Gust I. D. Control of hepatitis B in Australia. The case for alternative strategies. *Med J Aust* 1992; 156: 819–21.

2 National Health and Medical Research Council. Hepatitis B. In: *The Australian Immunisation Handbook*. 7th edn. Canberra: Australian Government Publishing Service, 2000, pp. 118–33.

3 Lau J. Y. and Wright T. L. Molecular virology and pathogenesis of hepatitis B. *Lancet* 1993; 342: 1335–40.

4 European Consensus Group on Hepatitis B Immunity. Are booster immunisations needed for lifelong hepatitis B immunity? *Lancet* 2000; 355: 561–5.

5 Zuckerman J. N., Sabin C., Craig F. M., Williams A. and Zuckerman A.J. Immune response to a new hepatitis B vaccine in health care workers who had not responded to standard vaccine: randomised double blind dose-response study. *Br Med J* 1997; 314: 329–33.

6 Mahoney F. J., Stewart K., Hu X., Coleman P. and Alter M. Progress toward the elimination of hepatitis B virus transmission among health care workers in the United States. *Arch Intern Med* 1997; 157: 2601–5.

25 | HIV testing in Australia

A. M. Breschkin, C. J. Birch and M. G. Catton

Introduction

Testing for HIV infection in Australia is delivered by way of a three-tiered system. Blood banks and approved public and private laboratories undertake screening tests to detect antibodies to HIV, and blood banks have recently also commenced nucleic acid testing (NAT) for viruses including HIV as an additional safeguard to protect the blood supply. Reactive specimens are referred by these laboratories to a state reference laboratory (SRL) for confirmatory testing. SLRs also undertake monitoring of HIV antiviral therapy with quantitative NAT, and have begun to introduce testing for HIV antiviral drug resistance. The National Serology Reference Laboratory (NRL) has the responsibility to evaluate new diagnostic tests, provide additional confirmatory tests, and to develop a consensus on the interpretation of results. In collaboration with the SLRs the NRL also distributes proficiency panels for HIV antibody testing and nucleic acid testing.

Serological testing

In Australia the most widely used HIV antibody screening assays are enzyme immunoassays (EIA). A positive test occurs when antibodies in the test serum bind to purified HIV antigens coating a test well or bead, in the presence of antibodies to human globulin chemically linked to an enzyme, or in some test formats to enzyme-labelled HIV antigen. The presence of the bound HIV antibody/antiglobulin antibody complex is detected by enzymatic cleavage of an appropriate substrate to yield a colour reaction. The sensitivity and specificity of the current generation of HIV screening EIA assays is extremely high. Currently, the rate of repeatably reactive test results in sera from healthy uninfected individuals is between 0.05% and 0.20%, depending on the source of antigen and the format of the test.

In 1993, combined screening tests for HIV-1 and HIV-2 antibodies were introduced in Australia. To date there have been only four confirmed cases of HIV-2 infection in Australia. Supplemental assays which discriminate HIV-1 and HIV-2 serological reactivity are used by reference laboratories. In 1999 screening assays with enhanced detection of the highly divergent HIV-1 Group O variants were introduced in Australia. Group O strains have been isolated from AIDS patients infected in Cameroon, but have not been reported in Australia to date.

Sera found to be repeatedly reactive by HIV screening tests are referred to a SLR for confirmatory testing by Western blot assay. In this assay, HIV-specific antibodies from test serum bind to the major structural proteins of the HIV-1 virus (see Fig. 25.1 on page 164) immobilised as distinct bands on a strip of nitrocellulose paper or nylon.

Much of the HIV virion's envelope protein is comprised of cell-membrane-derived material. Virus-specific glycosylated proteins in the envelope are gp120 and the transmembrane protein gp41, both of which originate from the same precursor protein. Specific amino acid sequences on gp120 determine cell tropism in vivo. The matrix protein p17 lies directly below the envelope. The core protein p24 is external to the ribonucleoprotein p7, which is itself closely associated with the viral nucleic acid (RNA). The presence of two copies of RNA in each virion is an essential prerequisite for the reverse transcription process, which is carried out by the HIV reverse transcriptase (RT) (p66) and involves the conversion of viral RNA to DNA. The HIV DNA is integrated into the cell genome as proviral DNA through the activity of the integrase (p32). Many of these viral components can be detected using assays available to the laboratory. The Western blot assay is

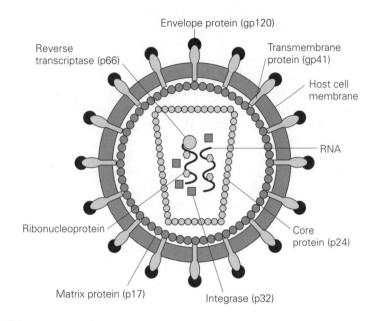

FIGURE 25.1 The HIV virion

capable of detecting antibodies to both structural and non-structural (enzymes) proteins. Nucleic acid assays can detect DNA following reverse transcription and quantitate the number of copies of RNA present in virions within the blood and other body fluids.

In a Western blot assay, detection of bound anti-HIV antibodies is achieved using an enzyme labelled anti-human globulin antibody and enzyme substrate as described above for EIA. Each protein is located at a different position on the Western blot strip and the appearance of a dark band at that site indicates the presence of antibody to a particular component of the virus. The commercial Western blot used in Australia also includes an HIV-2 specific peptide which reacts with HIV-2 positive sera. An HIV-2 Western blot is available at the NRL to confirm suspected HIV-2 infections.

According to current Australian guidelines, a serum is considered positive for HIV antibodies if it is repeatedly reactive on an HIV screening assay, and displays reactivity on a Western blot to at least one envelope glycoprotein and at least three other viral specific proteins. Sera which produce bands not fulfilling the positive criteria are reported as indeterminate. Indeterminate sera may represent partially complete seroconversion during acute HIV infection, or spurious reactivity not associated with HIV infection. These may be distinguished by the profile of bands present, together with follow-up of individuals who have profiles associated with high likelihood of early HIV infection. The indeterminate profiles are grouped as follows:

- Group 1: reactivity to viral proteins but not including p18, p24, or any envelope glycoproteins
- Group 2: reactivity to viral proteins including p18, but not including p24 or any envelope glycoproteins
- Group 3: reactivity to viral proteins including p24, but not to any envelope glycoproteins
- Group 4: reactivity to envelope glycoproteins but to fewer than three other viral proteins.

Figure 25.2 (on page 166) shows a series of three Western blot strips, demonstrating seroconversion to HIV over a period of 6 weeks in a recently infected patient. The first specimen, obtained at the time of presentation with a febrile illness suspected to be acute HIV infection, was non-reactive in a screening EIA and gave no bands on a Western blot. HIV proviral DNA was detected by DNA polymerase chain reaction PCR in peripheral blood mononuclear cells from a specimen of anti-coagulated blood obtained at this time, and p24 antigen was detected in serum. The second specimen obtained 3 weeks later was reactive by screening EIA for HIV antibody, and gave a group 4 indeterminate pattern on the Western blot (gp160, gp120 and p24). The patient remained DNA PCR positive but p24 antigen was negative by this time. The final specimen, obtained 6 weeks after the first, was reactive by screening EIA and gave a fully positive Western blot. The patient remained positive by DNA PCR, and p24 antigen was again negative.

Experience has shown that indeterminate patterns which do not include antibodies to p24 or an envelope band (groups 1 and 2) are not uncommon in uninfected individuals and are extremely unlikely to represent HIV seroconversion. In the early stage of infection, at the time of seroconversion, antibody to core protein (p24) and/or the glycoproteins are the first markers to be detected, potentially giving rise to group 3 or 4 indeterminate patterns (see Fig. 25.2). For this reason, individuals whose sera produce these patterns should be monitored over a 12-week period for evidence of seroconversion. In most patients who are seroconverting, samples collected 4 weeks

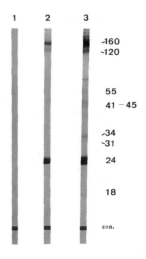

1	(Time of) presentation
2	3 weeks
3	6 weeks

FIGURE 25.2 A series of three Western blot assays demonstrating seroconversion to HIV over a period of 6 weeks in a recently infected patient

after the first demonstration of a group 3 or 4 indeterminate pattern will show progression to full Western blot positivity. After 12 weeks of follow-up effectively all acutely HIV infected individuals will have developed a positive Western blot. Those showing no progression after 12 weeks are reported as HIV-seronegative.

Sera repeatedly reactive on an HIV screening assay but displaying no bands on a Western blot may be reported as negative by many Australian reference laboratories. However it is our practice to retest such patients after a 4-week interval because the current EIA screening assays are more sensitive at detecting HIV antibodies during early seroconversion than the Western blot. Very rarely a serum with this pattern of reactivity represents the very early stages of HIV seroconversion. If no bands have appeared on a Western blot after 4 weeks, the possibility of early seroconversion is excluded, and we report the patient to be HIV seronegative.

The time between appearance of an infectious viraemia and seroconversion, the so-called 'infectious window period', has been estimated to be 22 days with current generation antibody tests.[1] Although cases of late seroconversion have been reported, their occurrence is rare, and it is difficult to determine whether these are genuine late seroconversions or represent subsequent exposures to the virus. Circulating p24 antigen and HIV nucleic acid may appear early in HIV infection during the antibody negative window. Assays for p24 antigen are usually positive for only a few weeks; p24 antigen then disappears (or declines to very low levels) until the onset of clinical AIDS at which stage it may become strongly positive. Since the introduction of nucleic acid-based assays in HIV diagnosis (see below), testing for p24 antigen has been largely superseded.

HIV culture

Virus isolation played an important role in the initial studies of HIV infection. However, the availability of HIV-specific nucleic acid detection and quantitation has, to a large extent, superseded this method as a means of detecting HIV early in infection and monitoring viral replication late in the disease process. Virus isolation remains important in evaluation of antiviral compounds, in the detection of antiviral drug resistant strains, and in the study of the pathogenesis of HIV infection.

Diagnosis of HIV-1 infection using nucleic acid tests

A strong case exists for the use of HIV nucleic acid testing to provide a diagnosis in situations where the utility of serology is limited but significant risk of HIV infection exists. Examples include early diagnosis of acute HIV infection, diagnosis of paediatric HIV infection in children less than 18 months of age, and occasional cases where full seroconversion is delayed by early intervention with antiretroviral therapy. Currently in Australia, the most frequent indication for HIV diagnostic nucleic acid testing is determination of HIV infection status prior to the appearance of HIV antibody to facilitate early antiretroviral therapy. Until the issue of the optimal time to commence antiretroviral therapy is resolved, a proportion of newly infected individuals may opt for early intervention with drugs. The increased sensitivity of molecular assays over serological techniques in early acute HIV infection provides the rationale for this to occur. In addition, early diagnosis of the HIV seroconversion syndrome, with appropriate counselling of the infected individual, may limit further transmission of the virus.

Consensus does not currently exist regarding guidelines for the use of HIV nucleic acid tests in diagnosis outside paediatric infection. In general, detection of proviral DNA in infected cells is considered the test of choice in diagnosis, while quantitative RNA assays are reserved for providing information on the likely progression of the disease and the response to antiretroviral therapy. A commercial proviral DNA PCR (Amplicor HIV-1, Roche Diagnostics) is available in Australia. For the time being, a positive Western blot using the criteria described above remains the definitive diagnostic test for HIV infection, and Western blot confirmation of presumptive nucleic acid test results should be obtained as soon as practically possible.

Measuring HIV viral load using nucleic acid tests

The availability of nucleic acid assays to quantitate HIV-1 in blood has had a significant impact on the management of infected individuals, particularly for prognostication, and monitoring the response to antiretroviral drug therapy. Several commercial assays are now available for this purpose in Australia, including the Amplicor HIV-1 Monitor (Roche Diagnostics), Quantiplex HIV RNA (formerly Chiron Corp., now Bayer) and NASBA-QT (Organon Teknica). The lower limit of detection of these assays varies from 400 (Amplicor and NASBA-QT) to 500 (Quantiplex) copies of the HIV RNA genome per mL of sample. With modifications to the procedure, lower limits of detection of 50 RNA copies per mL may be achieved (so-called 'ultrasensitive' assays). Such increased sensitivity may have a prognostic value in selected cases.

The technical strategies used by each of the HIV quantitation kit manufacturers vary somewhat. The Amplicor assay involves the extraction of RNA from virions present in patient plasma, followed by reverse transcription of this target RNA to generate complementary DNA (cDNA). This cDNA is enzymatically amplified by polymerase chain reaction (PCR) using primers specific for a small conserved region within the HIV Gag protein gene. Incorporation into the reaction of a known concentration of synthetic internal standard having identical primer binding sites to the target sequence on the cDNA enables quantitation of the final products. The Quantiplex assay requires the capture and immobilisation of extracted RNA using multiple primers specific for the HIV pol gene. Branched amplifier molecules (bDNA) are then hybridised to the target-probe complexes. A further hybridisation reaction involving multiple alkaline phosphatase probes allows quantitation of the final product in the presence of an appropriate substrate (dioxetane).

In general, these quantitative assays yield similar results when directly compared.[2] They are specific for HIV-1 strains classified as being in the M (major) subtype (no commercial assay for HIV-2 is available), and appear to be equally efficient in detecting and quantitating each of the HIV clades (A to I) within this subtype. They are also capable of quantitating HIV in sites other than blood, such as cerebrospinal fluid. In Australia, the performance of HIV RNA quantitation assays is regulated through participation by laboratories in quality assurance programs overseen by the NRL.

Antiretroviral drug resistance testing

Fifteen antiretroviral drugs are now available for the treatment of HIV infection. These drugs fall into the classes of reverse transcriptase (RT) or protease (PR) inhibitors. During HIV replication, errors in the reverse transcription process may generate potentially drug-resistant virus and these mutant strains may subsequently be selected when suboptimal levels of inhibitor are present. Experience has shown that to achieve maximal suppression of virus replication, and therefore to prevent the development of resistance, antiretroviral therapy should be used in combinations containing at least three drugs, which may include examples from one or both classes.

The presence of drug resistance mutations impacts on virological and clinical responses to therapy. The prospective VIRADAPT[3] and GART[4] clinical studies have demonstrated an improved virological response for periods of up to 12 months in patients who have had resistance testing carried out, compared to a control group. Drug resistance testing for both these studies was undertaken using genotyping (see below) of the viral protease and reverse transcriptase genes, a method within the capabilities of most HIV reference laboratories in Australia.

Currently, three methods have been described which fall into the category of antiretroviral drug resistance tests. These are phenotyping, genotyping and virtual phenotyping.

Phenotyping

In the context of drug resistance testing, phenotyping involves the exposure of replicating HIV to one or more of the drugs available clinically. The concentration of drug that inhibits viral replication in the absence of cellular toxicity is then determined. Because of the large number of drugs used clinically and the requirement for replicating virus (which in Australia necessitates the use of Physical Containment Level 3 facilities), routine phenotyping has become the preserve of a small number of specialist laboratories overseas.

Genotyping

Genotyping involves the direct sequencing of the PR and RT genes of the major HIV species present at the time of blood collection. Extraction of RNA from virions in the plasma, followed by reverse transcription and amplification of these genes, results in a product that can be sequenced. The amino acid sequence is then deduced from this nucleotide sequence, and interpreted with respect to the virion's likely drug susceptibility profile. This process of interpretation is not always straightforward, although the presence of well-characterised mutations can predict resistance to certain inhibitors. There is a need for a consensus approach to the interpretation of codon changes in HIV proteins targeted by antiretroviral drugs, and this is being achieved in Australia through participation of reference laboratories in quality assurance programs and clinical trials.

Virtual phenotyping

Virtual phenotyping is a novel procedure used to derive a drug susceptibility phenotype through comparison of locally generated PR and RT gene sequences from a virus with an unknown phenotype with a similar or identical sequence derived from an HIV strain for which the phenotype is known. The technology is not available in Australia at the present time unless patients are enrolled in specific clinical trials. Comparison of sequences is undertaken electronically through access to a large database of HIV strains with well-characterised phenotypes and corresponding sequences. However, further studies are required to determine the exact relationship between it and the actual phenotype.

The future

The combination of screening assays and Western blot for detection of HIV antibody provides sensitivity in excess of 99% and specificity greater than 99.5%. It is unlikely that any significant room for improvement exists in the accuracy or robustness of this diagnostic algorithm. Considerable potential for change exists in the relative emphasis on serological testing and direct viral detection by nucleic acid tests, however. Because of their low cost and relative simplicity, antibody screening assays are likely to remain the first-line tests for screening of the general population for HIV infection. However, the great sensitivity of nucleic acid tests during acute HIV infection, and their freedom from indeterminate results suggests that an increasingly prominent role as diagnostic and confirmatory tests for HIV is likely in future.

REFERENCES

1   Allain J. P. Genomic screening for blood borne viruses in transfusion settings. *Clin Lab Haem* 2000; 22: 1–10.

2   Schuurman R., Descamps D., Weverling G. J. et al. Multicenter comparison of three commercial methods for quantification of human immunodeficiency virus type 1 RNA in plasma. *J Clin Microbiol* 1996; 34: 3016–22.

3   Durant J., Clevenbergh P., Halfon P. et al. Drug-resistance genotyping in HIV-1 therapy: the VIRADAPT randomised controlled trial. *Lancet* 1999; 353: 2195–9.

4   Baxter J. D., Mayers D. L., Wentworth D. N. et al. A randomized study of antiretroviral management based on plasma genotypic antiretroviral resistance testing in patients failing therapy. *AIDS* 2000; 14: F83–93.

26 | Testing for *Helicobacter pylori*

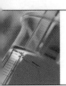

D. Badov

SYNOPSIS

Helicobacter pylori *commonly infects Australians and can cause gastritis, peptic ulcer disease and gastric cancer. Several non-invasive and invasive (requiring endoscopy) diagnostic tests are available. Non-invasive tests (breath tests or serology) are indicated when endoscopy is not required.*

Introduction

Helicobacter pylori is a spiral gram negative bacterium found in association with human gastric epithelial cells.[1] Infection of the gastric mucosa by *H. pylori* results in chronic antral gastritis and subsequently atrophic gastritis. Furthermore, *H. pylori* is a major pathogenic agent in duodenal and gastric ulcer disease, and has recently been implicated in gastric cancer and lymphoma. Seroepidemiological studies show that 30–40% of the Australian-born adult population are infected with *H. pylori*. The prevalence of infection is even higher in older age groups. The indications for *H. pylori* eradication and the optimal therapeutic regimen are still evolving.[1, 2] *H. pylori* can be detected using a range of non-invasive and invasive tests (Table 26.1).

TABLE 26.1 Properties of current clinical tests for *H. pylori*

	SENSITIVITY	SPECIFICITY	AVAILABILITY	COST (approx.)
INVASIVE				
Histology	95%	98%	A	$70
Culture	90%	100%	D	$32
Urease test	90%	95%	A	$1.80
NON-INVASIVE				
IgG serology	80–95%	80–95%	A	$14
14C or 13C urea				
breath test	95%	98%	A	$65
Stool antigen	95%	95%	D	$35

A = excellent, B = good, C = satisfactory, D = poor
Antibiotics, bismuth and proton pump inhibitors should be avoided during the
4 weeks before testing.

Technical aspects
Non-invasive tests
Breath tests
Several tests are based on the ability of *H. pylori* to produce urease.
This enzyme catalyses the degradation of urea to ammonia and
bicarbonate. In a breath test, urea that has been labelled with a
carbon isotope (13C or 14C) is swallowed. Infected patients rapidly
release labelled CO_2 into their breath. Carbon 14 can be easily
quantified using a scintillation counter. Carbon 13 has the
advantage of being non-radioactive, but requires more sophisticated
equipment for detection. Although the radioactivity of 14C appears
to be minimal, particularly with new protocols using 37 kBq
(1 microcurie) dosage, 13C breath tests should be used in pregnant
women and children. Breath tests have a sensitivity of about 95%
and a specificity of nearly 100%. The breath test usually becomes
negative within 1 month after eradication of *H. pylori* and is
particularly useful for assessing the efficacy of treatment.

Serology
H. pylori infection causes a local and a systemic immune
response. The presence of *H. pylori* can be shown by detecting
specific IgG and IgA antibodies in the serum. A number of
different serological tests are now commercially available and
used routinely in diagnostic laboratories. The sensitivity of these

tests is quoted as 80–95% and their specificity as 80–95%.[3]

Rapid office-based serological tests of serum/whole blood have recently become available. These tests have similar sensitivity and specificity to other serological tests and may be useful in diagnosing *H. pylori* in a primary care setting. The precise role of these tests in patients with dyspepsia presenting to general practitioners is currently being evaluated. Serology is not clinically useful for monitoring patients' post *H. pylori* eradication therapy as antibody titres may persist for many months.

Invasive tests

Invasive tests require upper gastrointestinal endoscopy and biopsy.

Histology

H. pylori causes chronic active inflammation within the gastric mucosa. Organisms can be seen on haematoxylin and eosin-stained biopsies as well as with special stains including modified Giemsa, Warthin Starry silver and acridine orange. In addition to the stain used, a second factor that influences the histologic detection of *H. pylori* is the uneven distribution of the organism through the gastric mucosa. Two antral biopsies are generally recommended. Sensitivity and specificity are approximately 95% and 98%.[4]

Culture

Culture from gastric mucosal biopsies is considered the gold standard of detection. Cultures are grown on selected and non-selected media at 35°C in a moist environment with CO_2 and hydrogen enrichment, and maintained for at least 7 days. Culture of the organisms is particularly useful in identifying the more pathogenic strains of *H. pylori* including cytotoxin production. In addition, antimicrobial sensitivity testing can be undertaken. The sensitivity and specificity of the test are approximately 90% and 100%. The sensitivity of this test is diminished if the number of organisms is small, culture techniques are inadequate, or if the patient has recently taken antimicrobial, bismuth or proton pump inhibitor therapy.

Because of the cost and the expertise required for culture of *H. pylori*, routine assessment is not currently recommended. The need for culture and sensitivity testing occurs in patients in whom initial eradication regimens fail.

Rapid urease test

Gastric mucosal biopsies can be inoculated onto a urea-containing medium and, if *H. pylori* is present, its urease splits the urea into ammonia and CO_2. The ammonia elevates the pH of the medium. This changes the colour of a pH-sensitive indicator. Commercially available agar-based tests such as CLO and HUT require up to 24 hours to become positive with about 70% positive within 2 hours. The sensitivity and specificity of urease tests are comparable to those of histology.

Diagnostic strategies

The test(s) employed depend on the patient's age, suspected diagnosis, previous diagnoses and treatment, the need for gastroscopy, local test availability and resources. Table 26.2 summarises potential approaches to the use of diagnostic testing.

TABLE 26.2 Clinical disease and *H. pylori* testing

INDICATIONS	TEST
DYSPEPSIA	
Children/pregnant women	Serology
	13C urea breath test
Young adults < 45 years old	Serology
	Urea breath test
Young adults with suspected malignancy or Barrett's oesophagus	Gastroscopy and biopsy
Older adults > 45 years old	Gastroscopy and biopsy
DUODENAL ULCER	
–current	Gastroscopy and biopsy
–previously documented	Urea breath test
GASTRIC ULCER	
post-treatment	Gastroscopy and biopsy
POST-*HELICOBACTER* TREATMENT	
Indication for gastroscopy (e.g. complicated ulcer, gastric ulcer)	Gastroscopy and biopsy
No indication for gastroscopy	Urea breath test
Failed eradication	Gastroscopy and biopsy culture and antibiotic sensitivity

Summary

H. pylori infection can be detected by several methods. The choice of a particular test depends on clinical factors, including the need for upper gastrointestinal endoscopy and monitoring of eradication therapy, availability, relative specificity, sensitivity and cost of the test. In most cases, testing should be done only if there is intention to treat if infection is found.

REFERENCES

1 Helicobacter pylori: *Guidelines for Healthcare Providers*. 3rd edn. Australian Gastroenterology Institute, 1999.

2 Lambert J. R. and Badov D. Gastric acid-related disorders: GORD and peptic ulcer disease. *Aust Fam Physician* 1995: 24: 1889–96.

3 Schembri M. A., Lin S. K. and Lambert J. R. Comparison of commercial diagnostic tests for *Helicobacter pylori* antibodies. *J Clin Microbiol* 1993: 31: 2621–4.

4 Lin S. K. et al. A comparison of diagnostic tests to determine *Helicobacter pylori* infection. *J Gastroenterol Hepatol* 1992: 7: 203–9.

Hepatitis C: diagnosis and monitoring

D. J. Siebert, A. M. Breschkin, D. S. Bowden and S. A. Locarnini

SYNOPSIS

The diagnostic blood tests for hepatitis C virus (HCV) are the serological assays, which detect antibodies to HCV, and the molecular assays, which detect or quantify HCV RNA. Screening tests for antibodies are first done using serological tests such as enzyme immunoassay. The molecular assays can be used to confirm the diagnosis or monitor the response to antiviral therapy. Detection of HCV RNA in patient serum provides evidence of active HCV infection. New assays can identify different HCV genotypes. All of these assays have limitations which affect their utility as diagnostic tests.

Introduction

Advances in viral diagnosis have significantly reduced the risk of post-transfusion hepatitis C in developed countries. The first serological assays were developed after the RNA sequence of hepatitis C virus (HCV) was identified in 1989.[1] Molecular biology techniques have since been used to detect and quantitate viral nucleic acid.

Various algorithms help the physician correctly identify patients infected with hepatitis C, evaluate them for the presence of significant liver disease and monitor their response to antiviral therapy. Interpreting hepatitis C tests depends on an awareness of the risk factors (Table 27.1) in conjunction with liver function test results.

TABLE 27.1 Risk factors for hepatitis C

Injecting drug use (past or present)
Blood or blood product use before May 1990
Abnormal liver function tests/cryptogenic liver disease
Occupational exposure to HCV
Extrahepatic conditions without apparent cause (e.g. mixed
    cryoglobulinaemia, acquired porphyria cutanea tarda, other syndromes
    linked to hepatitis C)
Imprisonment (past or present)
Renal dialysis
Tattoos, body piercing
Sharing razors and tooth brushes with HCV infected people‡
Migration from the Middle East, South-East Asia, Africa, South America*
Unspecified request for HCV testing (possible concealed risk)*
HCV infected parent (especially mother)‡
Sexual contacts of HCV infected people†

*   Potential or moderately increased risk only
†   Very low risk
‡   Low risk

Hepatitis C virus

Infectious HCV particles (virions) are less than 80 nm in diameter, have a lipid envelope and are strongly associated with the lipoprotein fraction of human serum. Each virion contains a single RNA molecule.

The virus circulates in the blood as a population composed of a master sequence and a large number of minor variants. This occurs because of random mutations during viral replication and also the selection pressure exerted by the host's immune response. This mixed population of viral particles is referred to as a quasispecies and is the basis of the variation found in the HCV genome. Such intrinsic variability may explain why chronic HCV develops in over 80% of acutely infected people. Comparison of HCV master sequences from around the world has led to subclassification of the virus into six distinct genotypes (HCV types 1 to 6).

Technical aspects
Hepatitis C serology

Anti-HCV screening assays

Enzyme immunoassay (EIA) is the most common method for detecting antibodies to HCV (anti-HCV). Three generations of anti-HCV screening assays have now been used in Australia. Improvements in the sensitivity of each successive generation of tests have been achieved by increasing the number of recombinant HCV antigens that are used, as well as modifying the other antigens present.

The drawback of the first generation tests was that they produced a high false-positive rate for anti-HCV in low-risk populations such as blood donors and people with no risk factors for HCV infection. They were also confounded by non-specific reactivity in patients with autoimmune diseases and hypergammaglobulinaemias. The sensitivity was also low because only one HCV antigen was included.

Supplemental assays

Supplemental assays for HCV antibodies are not widely used in Australian diagnostic laboratories. Such tests are designed to increase the specificity of serodiagnosis by detecting specific antibodies to individual HCV antigens.

All of the commercially available tests are expensive. Their cost effectiveness among various risk groups of patients has not been established. Their use is largely restricted to reference laboratories and the blood transfusion service. It has been argued that supplemental assays provide little useful information about samples that have already been found positive by current EIAs and that they contribute little to resolving weakly positive or discrepant results.

Sensitivity and specificity of serological assays

The overall sensitivity and specificity of second generation assays are both 95–98%. They may be increased somewhat by third generation tests which incorporate extra HCV antigens. The results obtained within each generation of tests are very similar, regardless of the commercial source of the test.

The results of screening tests can be divided into two sets based on the risk of infection:

1 low-risk populations, including blood donors and individuals with no risk factors for HCV infection
2 high-risk populations, including individuals with a risk factor(s) for HCV infection or documented liver disease presumed to be due to hepatitis C

Low-risk populations

The first generation tests suggested that between 0.3% and 1.5% of blood donors worldwide were positive for anti-HCV. In Australia, 0.45% of blood donors in New South Wales were found to be anti-HCV positive. At first, HCV was identified in only 95–98% of the units of blood responsible for post-transfusion hepatitis C infections. This suggested that some infected units of blood were being missed.

Second generation assays detected one additional anti-HCV positive donor per 1000 tested. However, the introduction of these two generations of tests led to successive reductions in the incidence of post-transfusion hepatitis. The third generation tests are thought to detect a single additional infectious unit of blood for every 10 000 units screened. Very recently, the Australian Red Cross Blood Transfusion Service has introduced nucleic acid amplification testing in order to detect HCV RNA (and human immunodeficiency virus RNA) in the blood of donors who may have been recently infected and not yet developed antibodies.

Now that screening assays are more sensitive, blood banks are more concerned with eliminating false positive screening results because their primary aim is to supply blood for transfusion which is verifiably HCV negative. The major problem in low prevalence groups, like blood donors, has been that 30–50% of sera found to be repeatedly reactive in first generation EIA screening tests could not be confirmed as positive by a supplementary antibody assay. With second generation EIAs, 39–50% of screen positive sera were later found to be false positives after supplementary antibody tests and nucleic acid assay.

High-risk populations

The vast majority of infected high-risk individuals are detected by the serological screening tests. However, first generation EIAs were only able to detect seroconversion in 50% of patients at 4 months and in 90% of patients 6 months after primary HCV infection. This relatively late seroconversion to non-structural viral antigens meant that a diagnosis was delayed or missed if patients were tested at the onset of acute hepatitis or too soon after exposure (Fig. 27.1).

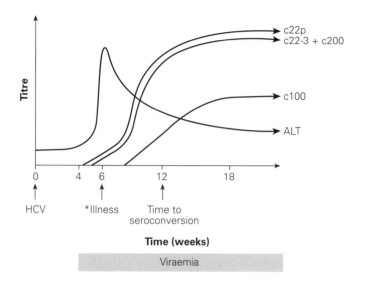

FIGURE 27.1 A graphic representation of antibody titre to HCV antigens versus time. ALT = alanine aminotransferase

Antibodies to the C100 antigen appear after the response to recombinant structural antigens such as c22p (third generation tests) and c22-3 (second generation tests). Symptoms (*) may develop in only 25% of cases.

Second generation EIAs overcame the problem of late seroconversion to anti-HCV positive status in infected patients. Between 12% and 20% of patients with chronic HCV who were not detected with first generation assays were seropositive after second generation tests. This seroconversion was usually detected within 12 weeks. A further 20% of patients with cryptogenic liver disease were also found to be anti-HCV positive by the new assays. Based on limited data, third generation tests appear to detect seroconversion earlier.

A minority of infected high-risk individuals may not become anti-HCV positive.[2] Immunosuppressed patients with defective lymphocyte responses may not produce detectable antibody. Furthermore, current antibody tests have been developed using recombinant antigens derived from HCV genotype 1 isolates. It has been shown that there is a lower sensitivity of detection of HCV non-genotype 1 infections compared to their genotype 1 counterparts. The sensitivity of all three generations of screening EIAs in high-risk groups is therefore slightly below that observed in low prevalence populations.

The Australian situation

In Australia, patients who have a positive screening test are most likely to have HCV if they have one of the following features:

- a past risk factor for HCV infection (e.g. past injecting drug use, tattoos)
- abnormal physical findings (e.g. hepatomegaly, excess spider naevi)
- elevated alanine aminotransferase (ALT) levels
- a positive polymerase chain reaction (PCR) for HCV in the blood.[3]

The most prevalent genotypes are 1, 3 and 2 (55%, 36% and 6% respectively). The currently used second- and third-generation screening tests do not appear to miss established infection in otherwise normal adults.[4] However, most published Australian data include individuals derived from both high-risk (diagnostic) and low-risk (blood donor) populations and do not distinguish between the two groups. In addition, rare high-risk patients who fail to seroconvert to anti-HCV positive status do not appear in the test performance statistics.

Clinicians should be aware that screening tests alone do not absolutely exclude hepatitis C in patients who have a risk factor for HCV or evidence of hepatitis. For example, in migrants from countries outside the U.S.A., Canada and northern Europe, infections due to other HCV genotypes (genotype 4-Middle East or genotype 6-South-East Asia) should be considered when there is clinical or biochemical evidence of hepatitis, but currently used HCV genotype 1 based screening tests are negative.

Diagnostic testing strategies

Under a new National Health and Medical Research Council (NHMRC) strategy, a positive test must be confirmed before a report will be issued.[5]

In blood donors, the aim of testing is to establish, with the greatest possible certainty, which donors are not infected. The NHMRC strategy advises blood banks to retest all positive sera in duplicate using the same screening EIA. If the repeat tests are both negative, the donation is considered HCV negative.[5] Clinical assessment will be required if the screening test is repeatedly positive.

For diagnostic laboratories, which are generally screening patients with liver disease or those who have a risk factor for HCV, the strategy aims to eliminate laboratory error and confirm the positive status of a reactive screening test (Fig. 27.2). Those sera which are positive in the first test are retested using a different EIA which contains a different range of recombinant HCV antigens. If the second test is positive, a positive result is issued to the clinician.

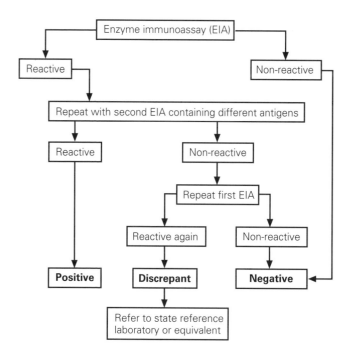

FIGURE 27.2 Recommended NHMRC protocol for HCV serology in diagnostic laboratories[5]

If there is a difference between the first and second test results, the serum is retested with the first EIA again. Where this repeat first test is no longer reactive, the screen is reported to the clinician as a true negative. However, if the repeat of the first EIA remains positive, the serum is referred to a reference laboratory for further testing.

Measuring viraemia

Molecular assays for viral RNA can be used to assess indeterminant EIA results. They can be divided into two distinct categories. The first and most common are qualitative tests which detect minute amounts of viral RNA in the serum, body fluids and tissues. These assays are based on the polymerase chain reaction (PCR) (see 'Diagnostic tests: DNA i. approach and techniques', *Aust Prescr* 1995; 18: 45–8). A positive result confirms the diagnosis of HCV infection; however, a negative result does not exclude infection.

Quantitative tests, including quantitative PCR and branch-chain DNA assays, have also been developed to measure HCV RNA levels in serum and other body fluids. These assays presently lack the sensitivity of the qualitative tests, but hold promise as a means of tailoring antiviral treatment schedules to pretreatment viraemia and for monitoring HCV replication during antiviral therapy.[6]

Qualitative tests

Detection of HCV RNA using reverse transcription polymerase chain reaction (RT-PCR) has become an increasingly important tool. The presence of HCV RNA in the serum differentiates current from past infection and can act as a marker of response to antiviral therapy. As most anti-HCV positive patients develop chronic hepatitis C, the NHMRC strategy suggests that testing for HCV RNA is not mandatory to confirm the presence of viraemia.[5]

Indications for qualitative PCR include:

- identification of viraemia to confirm active replication of HCV in people with equivocal or indeterminant serological tests (this includes newborns with passively acquired maternal antibodies and patients who are immunocompromised or immunosuppressed)
- early diagnosis of acute HCV infection
- monitoring during trials of treatments for HCV

- defining the route of transmission in epidemiological studies
- assessment of infectivity risk.[2]

When attempting to resolve equivocal and indeterminant serological profiles, the results of qualitative PCR assays vary with the characteristics of the population under test. For example, among screen-positive blood donors in the U.S.A., only 25% are positive by HCV PCR. The misdiagnosis of HCV on a single blood test should be avoided, especially in low-risk patients.

Quantitative tests

Before quantitative tests can replace qualitative tests, they must reach a higher degree of sensitivity.[6] Ideally, they should help us to answer these questions:

- Do HCV RNA levels predict the outcome of treated and untreated disease?
- What is the lowest level of HCV RNA indicative of hepatic viral replication and RNA clearance during therapy?
- Does the pretreatment RNA level predict clinically validated criteria of therapeutic response?

At this stage, we know that HCV RNA levels are relatively stable in untreated patients with chronic HCV and that interferon therapy reduces the viraemia in a significant proportion of treated patients.

Genotype assays

There is a high degree of variability among hepatitis C sequences obtained from different geographical sources and risk groups. These genotypes may have clinical significance. For example, some studies have shown that genotype 1b may be more likely to lead to cirrhosis and hepatocellular carcinoma.[7]

Genotyping has been used extensively in epidemiological studies. At present, its clinical utility as a predictor of the outcome of HCV disease is being evaluated in both treated and untreated patients. Using combination therapy of ribavirin and interferon, recent data show that treatment duration can be modified according to the infecting genotype of HCV. In patients infected with genotype 2 or 3, there is no need to continue therapy beyond 6 months. For patients infected with genotype 1, therapy needs to be extended for 12 months to achieve a higher sustained response rate.

Future trends

Diagnostic research will focus on several areas. One priority is the identification and production of better recombinant antigens to improve the detection of anti-HCV antibodies and enhance the specificity of both screening tests and supplementary assays. In addition, quantitative antibody assays may have a role in monitoring disease activity and response to therapy.

Improvements in the quantitative HCV RNA assays will be essential in the therapeutic monitoring of chronically infected patients and those undertaking antiviral therapy. The ability to detect and characterise genetic variants of HCV quickly will also become increasingly important. Variants that influence the virulence of HCV and the natural history of chronic hepatitis C, or confer resistance to new treatments, may have prognostic significance.

Summary

In Australian diagnostic laboratories, an anti-HCV screening test is reported as positive only after the patient's serum is found to be reactive in two different assay systems. While HCV RNA is likely to be present in the serum of high-risk patients who are anti-HCV positive, viral RNA is less likely to be detected in the serum of low-risk anti-HCV positive patients. Medium- to long-term follow-up, with repeated testing for evidence of viral RNA, may be required for those who do not have a risk factor for HCV infection, but who repeatedly test positive on HCV screening assays. Misdiagnosis of HCV on the basis of a single positive screening test should be avoided, particularly in low-risk patients. Quantitative assays and HCV genotyping may eventually provide data which predict the long-term risks and outcomes in both treated and untreated HCV infection.

REFERENCES

1   Choo Q. L., Kuo G., Weiner A. J., Overby L. R., Bradley D. W. and Houghton M. Isolation of a cDNA clone derived from a blood-borne

non-A, non-B viral hepatitis genome. *Science* 1989; 244: 359–62.

2 Gretch D. R. Diagnostic tests for hepatitis C. *Hepatology* 1997; 26 (3 suppl 1): 43S–47S.

3 Victorian Government Department of Human Services. *Management, Control and Prevention of Hepatitis C: Guidelines for Medical Practitioners*. Melbourne: Public Health Division, Victorian Government Department of Human Services, 1996.

4 McCaw R., Moaven L., Locarnini S. A. and Bowden D. S. Hepatitis C virus genotypes in Australia. *J Viral Hepat* 1997; 4: 351–7.

5 National Health and Medical Research Council. *A Strategy for the Detection and Management of Hepatitis C in Australia*. Canberra: Australian Government Publishing Service, 1997.

6 Pawlotsky J. M. Measuring hepatitis C viremia in clinical samples: can we trust the assays? *Hepatology* 1997; 26: 1–4.

7 Bruno S., Silini E., Crosignani A., Borzio F., Leandro G., Bono F., et al. Hepatitis C virus genotypes and risk of carcinoma in cirrhosis: a prospective study. *Hepatology* 1997; 25: 754–8.

FURTHER READING

Farrell G. C. Chronic viral hepatitis. *Med J Aust* 1998; 168: 619–26.

28 | Antinuclear antibodies

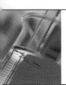

D. Barraclough

SYNOPSIS

The main use of the antinuclear antibody (ANA) test is in screening for multisystem autoimmune diseases, the prototype of which is systemic lupus erythematosus (SLE). However, antinuclear antibodies are sometimes found in a number of other conditions and in apparently healthy people.

Introduction

Antinuclear antibodies are directed against various antigenic components of nuclei in cells. The ANA is a broad screening test which, if positive, can be titrated and the pattern or likely specificity of the ANA observed. It is possible in appropriate circumstances to detect a number of antibodies targeted against specific nuclear antigens—that is, to determine the specificities of the ANAs more precisely.

Technical aspects

The usual method employs a cultured appropriately fixed human cell line (HEp-2 cells). These are prepared on slides and incubated with the patient's serum. The cells are then washed and if antinuclear antibody is present in the serum, it will adhere to the cell nuclei. The second stage is a further incubation of the slide with a fluorescein-labelled antiserum to human gamma globulin. If antinuclear antibody is present, then this antiserum will adhere to the patient's antibody at the sites where it is attached to nuclei and can subsequently be detected by fluorescent light microscopy. The antibody titre can be determined by serial dilution. In addition to this, the pattern of staining can be assessed (Table 28.1 on page 190). The ANA patterns serve as a guide to the clinician and laboratory as to which test to request next in an attempt to determine the ANA specificity. This has some value in disease association, but it is far less specific than identification of the specific antigen/antibody reaction (e.g. detection of antibodies to double-stranded DNA, or detection of antibodies to the very soluble components of the nucleus called extractable nuclear antigens). Multiple antibodies may be present in the serum and so different patterns of fluorescence may be observed at different serum titres.

What does a positive ANA screening test mean?

The main use of the test is in screening for multisystem autoimmune diseases, particularly SLE. ANA-negative SLE does occur but this is very uncommon and in such a case Ro* antibodies are usually present. In SLE, the ANA test will usually be positive in high titre. However, a positive ANA test may occur in a number of other conditions (Table 28.2 on page 190). Hence, the test is a good one for screening for SLE, although more specific tests are needed to confirm the diagnosis. It is important that, as for rheumatoid factor, the result is interpreted in conjunction with the other clinical and laboratory information.

Drug-induced antinuclear antibodies

Antinuclear antibodies may be induced in significant numbers of patients on certain drugs. These include hydralazine and procainamide particularly, and uncommonly with some other drugs. Only a small proportion of patients with ANAs induced by these drugs will go on to develop SLE. These ANAs are directed against histones and are usually associated with rheumatoid factor. Antihistone antibodies also occur in a minority (20–30%) of

TABLE 28.1 Patterns of immunofluorescence in antinuclear antibodies

HOMOGENEOUS
Homogeneous means the whole of the nucleus is evenly stained; this may be shiny or matt. This pattern may occur in many of the connective tissue diseases and in drug-induced systemic lupus erythematosus. A shiny homogeneous pattern suggests the specificity is anti-double-stranded DNA.

SPECKLED
There are many patterns of speckling ranging from 'diffuse grainy', which may be seen in scleroderma, to coarse speckles representative of the anti-Sm of systemic lupus erythematosus and the anti-Ul ribonucleoprotein of mixed connective tissue disease, to sparse discrete dots seen in primary biliary cirrhosis and many discrete dots seen in the anticentromere antibodies of limited cutaneous scleroderma. Often the specificities of speckled pattern ANAs are unknown and the disease associations not yet recognised.

NUCLEOLAR
The patterns within the nucleolus may be homogeneous, speckled or clumpy, each representing different specificities. About 50% of those patients with antinucleolar antibodies have scleroderma.

CENTROMERE
The dots seen in this pattern represent centromeres. The pattern occurs in about 90% of patients with the limited cutaneous (CREST) type of scleroderma and less commonly in other scleroderma patients.

MISCELLANEOUS
Several other patterns have been described which do not fit into the above classification. Anti-spindle, anti-mid-body, anti-lamin and anti-centriole patterns are some examples. Anti-proliferating nuclear cell antigen (PCNA) reacts only with the nucleus of dividing cells.

TABLE 28.2 Some conditions which may have a positive ANA test

Systemic lupus erythematosus (SLE)
Rheumatoid arthritis (RA)
Juvenile chronic arthritis
Primary Sjögren's syndrome
Scleroderma
Mixed connective tissue disease
Autoimmune chronic active hepatitis
Apparently healthy people (especially in the elderly)*
Some drug therapy, e.g. hydralazine, procainamide

---

* If the titre is high (≥ 1:640) it is advisable to review the case and repeat the test in 6 months' time.

patients with idiopathic SLE when these drugs are not implicated. Antibodies to double-stranded DNA are rarely detected in drug-induced SLE.

Identification of the specificities of ANA

A number of specific ANAs can be tested for by special techniques. These antibodies should not be looked for routinely, but are usually tested for when a positive ANA screening test result in significant titre (e.g. greater than 1:160) has been obtained in a patient thought to have a multisystem autoimmune disease associated with the specific antibody. Some are strongly suggestive of a particular disease, but in general results must always be interpreted in the context of the other clinical and laboratory data.

Some examples are:

■ *Antibodies to double-stranded (ds) DNA (DNA binding test).* The DNA binding test detects antibodies to ds DNA. It is requested when the clinical features suggest SLE and a positive ANA screening test, usually of homogeneous pattern, has been obtained. Although positive tests have been reported in several conditions other than SLE, it is a highly specific test, particularly if strongly positive. Positive results are present in approximately 60–70% of patients with active SLE.

■ *Antibodies to extractable nuclear antigens (ENA antibodies)*
  – *Antibodies to Sm.** This antibody is highly specific for SLE, but is present in only 4% of white Australians with SLE. It is found in about 30% of Asians with SLE. The ANA pattern is speckled.
  – *Antibodies to U1 ribonucleoprotein (U1 RNP).* These are found in mixed connective tissue disease (MCTD) (an illness often consisting of overlapping features of SLE, scleroderma and polymyositis), but may also occur in SLE, especially in Asians. The ANA screening test is positive with a speckled pattern in high titre.
  – *Antibodies to Ro* (SS-A).* These are found in Sjögren's syndrome, SLE and some other connective tissue diseases. The ANA may be either positive or negative, depending on how the HEp-2 cells are fixed. Neonatal SLE and congenital heart block are associated with maternal antibodies to Ro, although only a small proportion of women with these antibodies will have children who develop these problems.

- *Antibodies to La* (SS-B)*. As with antibodies to Ro, they may occur in primary Sjögren's syndrome and Sjögren's syndrome associated with SLE. The ANA is positive in speckled pattern.
- *Antibodies to Scl-70 (topoisomerase I)*. These antibodies are seen in approximately 20–30% of patients with scleroderma and are highly specific for scleroderma. The ANA is positive in speckled pattern.
- *Antibodies to Jo1**. These antibodies are seen in approximately 30% of patients with polymyositis. The ANA is negative.

* These antibodies were named after the first two letters of the surnames of the patients in whose serum the antibodies were first discovered.

Summary

The ANA test is a very sensitive test for the diagnosis of SLE but has low specificity, being positive in a number of other conditions and in some apparently healthy individuals. Positive results must always be interpreted in conjunction with other clinical information and sometimes more specific tests.

ACKNOWLEDGMENT

The author gratefully acknowledges the help of Dr Senga Whittingham of the Walter & Eliza Hall Institute in the preparation of this article.

Rheumatoid factor

29

D. Barraclough

Introduction

It was noted by Waaler in 1937 that a high proportion of sera from patients with rheumatoid arthritis agglutinated sheep erythrocytes sensitised with rabbit immunoglobulin G (IgG) antibodies to sheep erythrocytes. The term 'rheumatoid factor' evolved, and it has subsequently been found that rheumatoid factors are antibodies specific to antigenic determinants on the Fc fragments of human or animal immunoglobulin G (IgG). The rheumatoid factor commonly tested for is an immunoglobulin M (IgM), although immunoglobulins of several other classes have been demonstrated by special techniques.

Technical aspects

A number of different methods have been used. Whichever method is employed, it is important that a titre or some quantitative measure of the degree of positivity is obtained.

Latex test

Particles of polystyrene are coated with human IgG. Patients' sera containing rheumatoid factor will bind to the IgG and consequently precipitate the polystyrene particles. Serial dilutions are subsequently done.

Sheep erythrocyte agglutination (Rose Waaler test)

This test is rarely done now. Rabbits are immunised against sheep erythrocytes and the globulin from the rabbit serum obtained. This is subsequently used to coat sheep erythrocytes but not in sufficient quantities to agglutinate them. Patient's serum is then added to the sheep erythrocytes and, if rheumatoid factor is present, it will cause agglutination because of the reaction of the rheumatoid factor in the patient's serum with the IgG coating the sheep erythrocytes. Again, serial dilutions are done.

Nephelometric method

This is the method used routinely now. Nephelometry is a sensitive technique for measuring the degree of light scatter caused by the interaction of rheumatoid factor and heat-aggregated human IgG.

What does a positive test mean?

As well as in rheumatoid arthritis, rheumatoid factor can be detected in otherwise normal people and also in a number of other diseases (Table 29.1). These include other connective tissue diseases, some hepatic and pulmonary diseases, and also some infections. It is important to note that not all patients with rheumatoid arthritis have a positive rheumatoid factor test. Hence, the presence of a rheumatoid factor must be interpreted in the clinical context and not used as a diagnostic test in isolation.

Although of use in confirming a clinical diagnosis of rheumatoid arthritis, rheumatoid factor is of no use in following the course of the disease. If a significantly positive result has been obtained, there is no indication for serial measurements.

If a patient has a symmetrical inflammatory polyarthritis involving appropriate joints, if rheumatoid factor is present in high titre, and there is nothing on clinical or laboratory grounds to suggest an alternative diagnosis, then the patient almost certainly has sero-positive rheumatoid arthritis. A similar patient with a negative rheumatoid factor still probably has rheumatoid arthritis but it is important to check carefully that there are no

TABLE 29.1 Diseases which may be associated with a positive rheumatoid factor

CONNECTIVE TISSUE DISEASES	Rheumatoid arthritis
	Sjögren's syndrome
	Scleroderma
	Systemic lupus erythematosus
	Mixed connective tissue disease
INFECTIONS: VIRAL	Infectious mononucleosis
	Hepatitis
	Others
BACTERIAL	Tuberculosis
	Subacute bacterial endocarditis
	Leprosy
	Brucellosis
	Syphilis
	Bronchiectasis
PARASITIC	Malaria
MISCELLANEOUS	Some neoplasms
	Cryoglobulinaemia
	Chronic liver disease
	Sarcoidosis
	Chronic pulmonary fibrosis

features to suggest an alternative form of sero-negative inflammatory arthritis. Approximately 70% of patients with rheumatoid arthritis will have a positive rheumatoid factor, although this may take some months after the manifestation of clinical disease to become positive in some patients.

If the clinical picture is at all atypical for rheumatoid arthritis or is suggestive of some other condition (Table 29.1), then the rheumatoid factor may well be a 'false positive'. Low titre rheumatoid factor results are present in up to 10% of the elderly population.

Summary

A positive rheumatoid factor test in an appropriate clinical context may provide supportive evidence for the diagnosis of rheumatoid arthritis and does have some prognostic importance, tending to occur in more severe rheumatoid arthritis. However, 'false positives' do occur, and up to 30% of patients with rheumatoid arthritis remain sero-negative throughout the course of their illness. Hence, the result of a rheumatoid factor test should always be interpreted taking into account the clinical and other laboratory features.

Creatinine clearance and the assessment of renal function

30

B. J. Nankivell

SYNOPSIS

The selection of the most appropriate measurement of renal function depends on the clinical question being asked, the accuracy required and the inconvenience to the patient. Serum creatinine and calculated creatinine clearance yield a reasonable estimation of renal function with minimal cost and inconvenience. A urinary creatinine clearance is more accurate if the urine collection is complete. Isotopic measurement of glomerular filtration rate can be used when greater accuracy is required, when renal function is poor or muscle mass is significantly outside the normal range. Glomerular filtration rate should be corrected for body surface area and interpreted in the context of physiological effects such as pregnancy and blood pressure.

Introduction

Estimation of renal function is important in a number of clinical situations (Table 30.1 on page 198), including assessing renal damage and monitoring the progression of renal disease. Renal function should also be calculated if a potentially toxic drug is mainly cleared by renal excretion. The dose of the drug may need to be adjusted if renal function is abnormal.

**TABLE 30.1 Indications for renal function testing
(GFR = glomerular filtration rate)**

TEST	SETTING	CLINICAL INDICATION
SERUM CREATININE	Screening for renal disease	Hypertension Urine abnormalities Potential renal diseases (e.g. diabetes) Non-specific symptoms (e.g. tiredness)
	Monitoring renal function	Chronic renal disease Transplantation Drug toxicity
CALCULATED GFR/CREATININE CLEARANCE	Initial evaluation of renal disease	Glomerulonephritis Proteinuria Chronic renal failure Chemotherapy dosing
	Monitoring of renal disease	Glomerulonephritis Chronic renal failure
ISOTOPIC GFR	Accurate GFR	Monitoring therapy in glomerulonephritis
	Low levels of GFR	Deciding when to start dialysis Chronic renal failure
	Altered muscle mass	Body builder Renal impairment in a wasted patient

Renal function and glomerular filtration rate

The glomerulus is a high-pressure filtration system, composed of a specialised capillary network. It generates an ultrafiltrate that is free of blood and significant amounts of blood proteins. Renal damage or alterations in glomerular function affect the kidneys' ability to remove metabolic substances from the blood into the urine.

Glomerular filtration rate (GFR) is the rate (volume per unit of time) at which ultrafiltrate is formed by the glomerulus. Approximately 120 mL are formed per minute. The GFR is a direct measure of renal function. It is reduced before the onset of symptoms of renal failure and is related to the severity of the structural abnormalities in chronic renal disease. The GFR can predict the signs and symptoms of uraemia, especially when it falls to below 10–15 mL/min. Unfortunately it is not an ideal index, for it is difficult to measure directly, and is sometimes insensitive for detecting early renal disease.

Tubular function

Although glomeruli control the GFR, damage to the tubulointerstitium is also an important predictor of GFR and progression towards renal failure. Renal tubules make up 95% of the renal mass, do the bulk of the metabolic work and modify the ultrafiltrate into urine. They control a number of kidney functions including acid-base balance, sodium excretion, urine concentration or dilution, water balance, potassium excretion, and small molecule metabolism (such as insulin clearance). Measurement of tubular function is impractical for daily clinical use, so we usually use the GFR to assess renal function.

Normal range for GFR

The GFR varies according to renal mass and correspondingly to body mass. GFR is conventionally corrected for body surface area (which equates with renal mass), which in normal humans is approximately 1.73 m^2 and represents an average value for normal young men and women. When the GFR is corrected for body surface area, a normal range can be derived to assess renal impairment.

The normal corrected GFR is 80–120 mL/min/1.73 m^2, impaired renal function is 30–80 mL/min/1.73 m^2 and renal failure is less than 30 mL/min/1.73 m^2. The corrected GFR is approximately 8% lower in women than in men, and declines with age at an annual rate of 1 mL/min/1.73 m^2 from the age of 40.

In addition to ageing there are a number of physiological and pathological conditions that can affect GFR, including pregnancy, diabetes, hypertension, medications and renal disease. These conditions should be considered when interpreting a patient's GFR.

Measurement of GFR by renal clearance

The GFR cannot be directly measured in humans, but can be estimated from urinary clearance of a substance (x), given by the equation:

Urinary clearance $(x) = U_x V / P_x$

where U is the urinary concentration of an ideal filtration marker of x, V is the urine flow rate and P_x is the average plasma concentration of x.

An 'ideal filtration marker' is a substance that is freely excreted by glomerular filtration, without tubular reabsorption or secretion. The clearance of ideal filtration markers can be shown mathematically to be an accurate estimate of GFR.

The balance concept

The plasma concentration of a substance in a steady state depends on the balance of the input (from either endogenous production or exogenous intake) and the clearance from the blood (by either excretion or metabolism). When an ideal filtration marker is used (and there is no hepatic metabolism or non-renal clearance) and the input is constant (for example, by endogenous creatinine generation), then the plasma concentration is inversely proportional to GFR.

Methods to estimate GFR

GFR can be estimated from the serum concentration of filtration markers (such as creatinine or urea) or the renal clearance of these markers. Each method has its advantages and disadvantages in terms of accuracy, cost and convenience (Table 30.2).

TABLE 30.2 Assessment of renal function

METHOD	ACCURACY	COST	CONVENIENCE
Serum creatinine	**	$	***
Serum urea	*	$	***
Calculated creatinine clearance	***	$	***
Measured creatinine clearance	** to ***	$$	*
Isotopic glomerular filtration rate	****	$$$	*

Serum creatinine or calculated creatinine clearance are the two most convenient estimates of GFR, requiring only a single blood sample. Measured creatinine clearance requires a 24-hour urinary collection while isotopic methods involve intravenous injection of a nuclear tracer, and two subsequent blood samples to estimate clearance. Both these methods are more expensive and less convenient to the patient. Selection of the most appropriate test depends on the clinical question, the required accuracy and cost (Table 30.2).

Serum creatinine

Serum creatinine is commonly used to screen for renal disease or to investigate urinary sediment abnormalities, hypertension or non-specific symptoms such as tiredness. It is also used to monitor renal function after transplantation, in chronic renal disease, and in patients with glomerulonephritis taking disease-modifying therapy. Serum creatinine can also be used to monitor the effects of nephrotoxic drugs such as gentamicin or anticancer drugs. Serum urea can be used to estimate renal function but is highly variable, less accurate and prone to errors.

Serum creatinine is mainly produced by the metabolism of creatine in muscle, but also originates from dietary sources of creatinine such as cooked meat. Creatinine generation from the muscles is proportional to the total muscle mass and muscle catabolism. In people with a relatively low muscle mass, including children, women, the elderly, malnourished patients and cancer patients, the serum creatinine is lower for a given GFR. There is a danger of underestimating the amount of renal impairment in these patients, as their serum creatinine is also relatively lower. For example, the GFR may be reduced as low as 20–30 mL/min in a small elderly woman, while her serum creatinine remains in the upper range of normal.

Creatinine is an imperfect filtration marker, because it is secreted by the tubular cells into the tubular lumen, especially if renal function is impaired. When the GFR is low, the serum creatinine and creatinine clearance overestimate the true GFR. Some drugs (such as cimetidine or trimethoprim) have the effect of reducing tubular secretion of creatinine. This increases the serum creatinine and decreases the measured creatinine clearance. Paradoxically, when these drugs are used, a more accurate measurement of GFR is obtained as it is largely free from the error contributed by the physiological tubular secretion of creatinine.

Calculated creatinine clearance

As serum creatinine is so highly dependent on age, sex and body size, a number of corrections and formulae have been developed to estimate the muscle mass and assumed creatinine production. The most well-known formula is the Cockcroft-Gault formula, which is relatively simple to use and reasonably accurate. It is given as:

Creatinine clearance (mL/min) =
(140 – age[years]) × weight(kg)/serum creatinine (micromol/L)
Multiply result by 1.22 for male patients.

This is a good estimate of GFR, but it becomes inaccurate when a patient's body mass is significantly outside the normal range (for example, morbid obesity or severe malnutrition) or when renal function is very impaired (i.e. GFR < 20 mL/min). In these circumstances an isotopic method can be used if the GFR needs to be accurately measured.

Creatinine clearance

Creatinine clearance has been used for many decades to estimate GFR. It involves a 24-hour urine collection to measure creatinine excretion. As the same sample can be used to measure the protein excretion rate, creatinine clearance is often used for the initial evaluation of renal diseases, such as glomerulonephritis. It can also be used to monitor the progression of chronic renal failure, the response to therapy or to help decide when to start dialysis in patients with declining renal function.

The major problem with measuring creatinine clearance is that the collection may be incomplete; often urine is passed into the toilet rather than into the collection bottles. This results in an underestimation of renal function, and has led some commentators to recommend alternative measures such as calculated creatinine clearance or an isotopic GFR. In hospital, especially when the patient is catheterised, creatinine clearance provides an accurate estimate of GFR. Overestimation of GFR occurs at low levels of renal function, due to tubular secretion of creatinine. This can be corrected by collecting the urine while the patient is taking cimetidine or by averaging a urea and creatinine clearance in a single 24-hour collection. To accurately define GFR at low levels of renal function, an isotopic GFR is recommended. (See Table 30.3.)

TABLE 30.3 Errors in measurement of renal function using creatinine

	EFFECTS ON CREATININE CLEARANCE	EFFECTS ON SERUM CREATININE
ASSAY INTERFERENCE		
Ketosis	Nil	↑
Hyperbilirubinaemia	Nil	↑
Cephalosporin	Nil	↑
INHIBITION OF TUBULAR SECRETION OF CREATININE		
Cimetidine or trimethoprim	↓*	↑
ALTERATION OF CREATINE/ CREATININE LOAD		
Eating cooked meat	↑	↑
Low protein diet	↓	↓
Body building	Nil	↑
Muscle wasting	Nil	↓
RENAL DISEASE	↓	↑

* Becomes more accurate at low levels of GFR when increased tubular secretion of creatinine is blocked.

Isotopic GFR

Isotopic GFR is the most accurate measurement of GFR, especially at low levels of renal function or with alterations of muscle mass. The most common isotopic marker is technetium 99m DTPA, given as a single injection. Two plasma samples are taken at 1–3 hours after injection. The GFR is calculated from the plasma clearance of the isotope. Isotopic GFR can be used for monitoring renal function over time, or in chronic renal failure patients approaching dialysis. Patients are usually tested every 2 to 5 years, because of the cost and inconvenience of the procedure.

Summary

Renal function can be evaluated by measuring the GFR. As it is not easy to measure the GFR directly, the serum creatinine concentration is often used to assess renal function. Creatinine clearance provides a more accurate assessment and can be calculated from the serum creatinine or more exactly from the results of a 24-hour urine collection. Isotopic methods can be used if a very accurate measurement of GFR is required.

Drug screens

31

N. A. Buckley

SYNOPSIS

The two types of drug screens are rapid tests and specific assays. Rapid tests are for a restricted range of substances (usually just drugs of abuse) and have limited sensitivity and specificity. When there are important medicolegal considerations, the results must be confirmed by more specific assays. Specific assays are labour-intensive tests that can detect most drugs but take much longer to perform. They are required where the concentration of the drug may lead to specific interventions (such as in certain overdoses). Conversely, even the most comprehensive negative screen cannot entirely rule out drug ingestion as some substances are difficult to detect. The knowledge of the laboratory staff should be utilised when ordering and interpreting the tests.

Introduction

'Drug screens' are simply tests for a range of drugs or other substances. They have a wide variety of uses and almost any bodily fluid can be screened. Routine use of drug screens does not improve clinical outcomes, but selective use may assist patient management and occasionally yield an unexpected diagnosis.

Types of drug screens

There are two main types of drug screens. Immunoassays screen for a limited range of selected substances. These assays are relatively quick and some can even be performed at the bedside. They are commonly used to detect drugs of abuse or to test for commonly ingested substances in overdose. There may be cross-reactivity with some chemically related substances and the test cannot detect uncommon or unsuspected drugs. Different brands of immunoassays have different problems with sensitivity and specificity. These problems should be outlined in the product information of the assays.

The second form of drug screening involves chromatography with or without mass spectrometry. This can detect most substances that are present in significant concentrations. Testing is relatively expensive and depends heavily on the skill and experience of the laboratory staff. Unless only specific substances are of interest, the turnaround time varies from days to weeks, so these tests are less likely to influence the acute management of a patient.

Screening tests most commonly use urine, but serum can also be used. In forensic studies, vitreous humour, pleural effusions, hair, bone or nails may be screened. Saliva, breath, sweat, and breast milk can also be screened when looking for drugs of abuse.

Indications for screening

Overall, screening is most frequently used in medicolegal situations. These include determining cause of death; detecting performance-enhancing drugs in athletes, and detecting drug abuse in the workplace; drug and alcohol rehabilitation programs; or for psychiatric patients. In most cases, detecting a drug, in any concentration, gives sufficient information.

In acute poisoning and other toxicological screening the drug concentration may be important so screening the urine may not be the appropriate investigation. Drug screens of the urine do not reveal the amount of drug or the time it was taken because the urinary concentration correlates poorly with serum concentrations. Detecting the presence of a drug does not tell you if it is at a toxic concentration or explain the clinical status of the patient. In these circumstances, serum may be a better body fluid to screen. This is particularly so for substances such as paracetamol, salicylates, anticonvulsants, alcohol, ethylene glycol, methanol, lithium and theophylline as their concentrations determine the treatment. In these situations specific assays are usually more appropriate than a 'drug screen'. Paracetamol is so commonly taken in overdose that a routine specific assay in unconscious patients is generally warranted. However, routine specific assays for other substances are not indicated unless there are signs or biochemical changes that raise suspicion of their ingestion. Quantitative screening for drugs is also important in patients with suspected brain death.

Technical aspects

To optimise the usefulness and the cost-effectiveness of drug screens there are several important factors. These include selection of a screening test appropriate to the patient, correct collection of samples, communication with the laboratory and follow-up tests where appropriate.

Selection of an appropriate screen

The most common clinical reason for requesting a drug screen is suspected ingestion of an unknown substance or substances. Examples include suspicions of overdose (e.g. coma, seizures, acidosis), malingering or child abuse (e.g. unexplained hypoglycaemia or ataxia), or illicit drug abuse (e.g. psychosis, mood swings). Where possible, the drug screen should relate to the patient's clinical presentation. For example, a patient with severe acidosis may be suspected of taking a number of substances. However, most immunoassay techniques do not detect many of the drugs and poisons that lead to acidosis. They are designed to detect only commonly used drugs of abuse and drugs that lead to coma, such as alcohol, benzodiazepines, opiates, amphetamines, tricyclic antidepressants, LSD, cocaine and marijuana. A 'negative' drug screen of the urine in a patient with acidosis would be largely unhelpful or misleading. Specific screening of the serum for ethylene glycol, methanol and salicylates, and chromatography to detect other unusual substances, may be quicker and much more useful investigations.

In many cases drug screens are done for legal or quasi-legal purposes and the screen must accurately detect substances relevant to that purpose (for example, drugs that might impair driving). Testing for other substances is irrelevant.

Communication with the laboratory

Most laboratories performing drug screens do large numbers of tests for non-clinical reasons. If you anticipate that the drug screen may alter your clinical management it is important to discuss the case with the laboratory. A history of the drugs the patient is known to take will help the laboratory to identify the substances you are not concerned about. Knowing which specific substances are suspected on clinical grounds helps the laboratory to tell you whether or not it can identify such substances, for how long they can be detected after ingestion and whether serum or urine is preferred. The laboratory may also alter the methods used to prepare the sample to maximise the sensitivity of the testing for those substances.

Collection of sample and follow-up tests (medicolegal cases)

Correct and explicit identification of the patient and sample, prevention of tampering during collection and a secure chain of custody are very important in medicolegal cases. If the result has important medicolegal implications the accuracy of the result should be confirmed by using more specific and accurate methods such as gas or liquid chromatography and mass spectrometry. Depending on the drug involved these tests are done on the same specimen or a different specimen.

False positive results

The most common cause of false positive results in clinical settings is the therapeutic use of barbiturates, benzodiazepines and/or opiates for sedation, anaesthetic induction or analgesia. Many immunoassays do not differentiate between drugs in these classes and may cross-react with related therapeutic substances. For example codeine (and poppy seeds) may lead to positive opiate reactions, and decongestants such as pseudoephedrine and phenylpropanolamine may lead to positive amphetamine reactions. Only discussion with the laboratory and further specific testing can clarify such results.

False negative results

False negatives can relate to the time of sampling (too soon or too late), the body fluid tested or the method used. Immunoassays test for a restricted range of chemically related substances. Even within pharmacological drug classes they may not detect substances that have identical effects but an unrelated chemical structure. For example, most immunoassays for opiates do not detect the structurally unrelated methadone, dextromethorphan or pethidine. Metals (e.g. mercury, arsenic) are not detected by the commonly used drug screens and require specific tests. Some toxic substances (insulin, succinylcholine, potassium) cannot be detected by any method, as any avid reader of crime fiction knows.

Other problems of interpretation

The detection of one substance does not exclude the presence of others which cannot be detected by the same method. Drugs with similar chemical structures, but different toxicities, may give the same result. For example, within the drugs in the amphetamine class (methamphetamine, MDMA, PMA, fenfluramine and pseudoephedrine) there is a non-overlapping spectrum of peripheral and central nervous system stimulant effects and serotoninergic effects which lead to quite different toxicological syndromes. Failure to appreciate that some positive immunoassay screens for amphetamines could indicate ingestion of any or all of these drugs may lead to inappropriate management.

Summary

Drug screens are a useful clinical tool if you are selective in their use, have realistic expectations of their sensitivity and specificity, and discuss the clinical setting and suspected drugs with the laboratory staff. Otherwise you may be better off disposing of the urine in the traditional and less expensive manner.

FURTHER READING

Eskridge K. D. and Guthrie S. K. Clinical issues associated with urine testing of substances of abuse. *Pharmacotherapy* 1997; 17: 497–510.
Braithwaite R. A., Jarvie D. R., Minty P. S., Simpson D. and Widdop B.

Screening for drugs of abuse I: Opiates, amphetamines and cocaine. *Ann Clin Biochem* 1995; 32: 123–53.

Simpson D., Braithwaite R. A., Jarvie D. R., Stewart M. J., Walker S., Watson I. W. et al. Screening for drugs of abuse II: Cannabinoids, lysergic acid diethylamide, buprenorphine, methadone, barbiturates, benzodiazepines and other drugs [review]. *Ann Clin Biochem* 1997; 34: 460–510.

Skelton H., Dann L. M., Ong R. T., Hamilton T. and Ilett K. F. Drug screening of patients who deliberately harm themselves admitted to the emergency department. *Ther Drug Monit* 1998; 20: 98–103.

Index

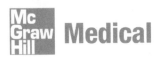

McGRAW-HILL MEDICAL PUBLISHING

McGraw-Hill has a well-established and extensive list of medical and health products that covers a wide range of medical disciplines for students, academics, practitioners and health workers. McGraw-Hill acquired Appleton & Lange to compliment and expand its collection and it has since strengthened its position at the fore of medical publishing.

OTHER RELATED MCGRAW-HILL TITLES

Birkett, Donald J., *Australian Prescriber's Pharmacokinetics Made Easy*

Guy, Duncan, *McGraw-Hill's Pocket Guide to ECGs*

Hancox, Bob & Whyte, Ken, *McGraw-Hill's Pocket Guide to Lung Function Tests*

Nicoll, Diana et al, *Pocket Guide to Diagnostic Tests 3rd edition*

Nigon, Donna L., *Clinical Laboratory Management: Management Leadership Principles for the 21st Century*

If you would like more information about other medical and health titles you may access the McGraw-Hill website on http://www.mghmedical.com.

To order McGraw-Hill products or receive a copy of the McGraw-Hill medical catalogue, please contact:

Product Manager, Medical
McGraw-Hill Australia Pty Limited
Level 2, 82 Waterloo Rd
North Ryde
NSW 2113
Australia

Tel: 61 2 9900 1854
Fax: 61 2 9878 8918
Em: cservice_sydney@mcgraw-hill.com